CRYSTALS

FOR BEGINNERS

THE ULTIMATE GUIDE TO UNDERSTAND THE HEALING POWER OF CRYSTALS

Table of Contents

INTRODUCTION

A crystal is a strong material comprising several molecules that develop in a repetitive, extremely unified model and then form a crystal lattice that spreads development in all directions.

The method of crystallization starts at the stage where the mantle of the earth and the crust meet. This extremely pressurized area with raging temperatures produces a liquid that flows into the fractures and cavities that have formed in the crust of the earth. As liquids cool minerals start to crystallize. This method requires time and is often hammered by broken sections, shifts in the setting, heat or strain. This can disrupt the development cycle and provide us with many of the incredible inclusions, phantoms, or healing fractures that we see today. Millions of years ago, natural disasters, weathering or erosion will bring the rocks nearer to the earth's surface to be found.

Crystals are one of nature's most organized and stable structures. Humans, on the other side, are complete opposites, meaning that we are prone to disorder and disease. Due to the crystalline structure, crystals have an incredible capacity to react to the stresses in their surroundings and to oscillate and emit particular vibrational energies and frequencies that beings naturally resonate and react to.

Crystal healing is the interplay between the domain of human energy and crystal energy. The active personal characteristics of crystals are harnessed by the physician in the healing process by tapping into the crystal vibration that is then used to integrate and repair the natural energy domain.

Crystals in History

The use and awareness of crystals and their powers have been common knowledge in ancient days.

The use of crystals in places of worship, shrines or sacred sights around the globe is well recorded by scientists and archeologists. More than just decoration, most ancient people celebrated the healing powers of crystals carried on the body and their capacity to grow the mind and provide transcendent experiences during celebrations or in private meditations.

For many societies, such as the Atlantis crystals, their existence was integral. Legend argues that crystals produced energy for entire towns and kept sacred information that was programmed into bits of transparent quartz and brought down through the centuries, enabling their culture to thrive.

The Egyptians were said to have constructed the Great Pyramid of Giza out of Granite, realizing that this mineral can produce electricity. Understanding that when granite is subjected to stress or power vibration, small quartz droplets produce electrical currents recognized as the piezoelectric impact (Darin, 2014). Prescient and semi-precious stones had a strong presence throughout their churches and sarcophagi and were constantly embellished with jewelry and headpieces to help to heal, reinforce management, provide security and improve power.

Ancient Indian groups thought that rocks such as rubies, sapphires and moonstones had strong associations to stars and planets. Astrological records dated as soon as 400 BC included descriptions of the strength of multiple rocks to counteract the negative impacts of planetary locations.

Ancient China thought that clear quartz would provide excellent spiritual enlightenment and that it was extremely sought after. They also regarded Jade to be the rock of heaven, carved into a multitude of mythical creatures as exhibits in households and sacred attractions. To this day, Jade stays one of the most famous rocks offering excellent luck and health to the proprietor.

In many of their healing rituals and circles, the Native American Indians used jewels and rocks. Turquoise was used to ward off evil spirits and alert the proprietor to potential risk. The Vikings used the energy of the crystals to safeguard them during their journeys, through conflicts and to guide them in navigation, while the Aztecs and the Mayans used the crystals as a medical diagnostic instrument.

CHAPTER 1
WHAT IS A CRYSTAL
AND HOW DOES IT FORM

Crystals are beautiful rock formations that have astounded people for thousands of years. They're used in many ways, not only as decorations. Years ago, radios were projected to make use of crystals to convey radio waves. Some instruments, such as quartz watches, still use crystals to this day. They have always been seen as something of value and are often put inside parts of jewelry with diamonds or other jewels. Most of the crystals are now human-made in laboratories. They are highly uncommon to be found on Earth.

What Are Crystals?

Crystals are nothing more than a fixed set of molecules or atoms. Crystals come in many different shapes and sizes and each has different features. What they're produced of determines how it's going to be formed. Some shells can be produced of salt— they create cubed crystals. Many are composed from other elements and shape entirely different forms. Examples of these are diamonds or rubies. There are some components that could produce more than one form. When the carbon element is in the form of a diamond, it can be used to cut gemstones, but we use it on a daily basis, in different manners. The most important way we use it is to deliver electricity to our homes and companies.

How Crystals Are Formed

If you would like to understand how crystals are formed, you can experiment in your own kitchen and see crystals forming with your own eyes. This can be achieved by placing a tiny quantity of table salt in some standard tap water, waiting for 24 hours and you'll see some beautiful cubed structures. This occurs because water evaporates, which allows the atoms that compose the salt (mineral) and water to grow nearer together. Eventually they're going to create a good little uniform bunch of atoms. The more they can come together, the more the structure becomes noticeable to the naked eye. Scientists can determine what mineral they're looking at by the way crystals are formed.

Not all the crystals are formed in the water. Many are crystallized in carbon. However, all crystals shape the same manner; atoms come together and become a group of uniforms. The process could take from a few days to maybe a thousand years. Natural crystals coming from Earth are the same thing. These crystals were formed in the crust of the Earth over a million years ago. They happen when the liquid in the earth is consolidated and the temperature chills. Other crystals shape when the liquid passes through the cracks and disperses the minerals into the cracks.

Interesting Facts on Crystals

Even without realizing, we use or see crystals often - salt, sugar, gemstones and snowflakes. Crystals are valued for their beauty of gemstones and appreciated for being useful in many electronic products. Some individuals also think that crystals have spiritual and healing characteristics. Their organized, repeated models are a marvel of nature and chemistry.

Types of Crystals

Crystals can shape in many forms, from simple cubic constructions to hexagonal or double pyramids to large spires with up to 10 or more sides. Some of them are not symmetrical from one hand to the other. The form of the crystal structure is determined by its chemical components and chemical bonds. Sometimes the crystalline structure shifts to the liquid state and becomes a liquid crystal often used in the present technology.

Common Crystals

Quartz is a crystal that many people understand. It develops in six-sided boxes and can come in a variety of colors, based on the chemical impurities in the column. An amethyst gemstone is a quartz form with chemicals that offer it a wealthy purple color. Table salt is a crystal formed by two chemicals, sodium and chloride, which come together in a cube-shaped crystalline structure. Epsom salts, used for healing, are produced of magnesium and sulfur and form a spicy, crystal-clear shape.

Where Crystals Come From

Natural crystals are dug out of the ground, where the temperature and stress of the earth lead them to form. Many crystals are also produced in laboratories under monitored circumstances for particular reasons.

Uses for Crystals

Quartz crystals have a natural property called piezoelectricity, the capacity to produce an electrical field that makes them very helpful in radio and video machinery. Silicon crystals are used to make chips that power our computers and photovoltaic cells used in solar technology. Crystals are often sliced and polished into jewels used in jewelry. Crystals are often used as ornamental artifacts and focal points for meditation and healing.

Make Your Own Crystals

At home, you can form your crystals. You'll need a heat-resistant glass container, a measuring cup, 1/2 cup of salt, 1 cup of cooking water, a pencil, a paper clip, a cotton cord, a spoon and a paper towel.

Tie the stick to one side of the pencil and the other end of the paper clip. Place your pencil across the bottom of your container. The cable is scarcely supposed to let the paper clip reach the ground. Boil 1 cup of water and add it to the container. Add 1/2 cup of salt to the water, one teaspoon at the moment. Stir in the water for each teaspoon until it dissolves. If you discover some salt in the bottom of the bottle, you can avoid adding more. This implies that the solution is "supersaturated." Put a string and a paper clip in a bottle with a on top and cover with a paper towel. After two days, you'll see a lot of crystals forming along the paper clip and the cord.

How Does a Sugar Crystal Grow?

Place a small quantity of sugar on a surface where is easy to observe it. You will be able to see that it is made of millions of small crystals. Now, if you put the same quantity of sugar in water, what happens is that the small particles disintegrate shortly after the contact. If you want to recrystallize the sugar, you have to choose between the two following methods.

Evaporation Reaction

Sugar molecules are the most stable ones in the crystalline structure. If you leave the solution of sugar submerged in water exposed, the water will evaporate and the solution will become increasingly focused. As the water molecules vanish, the sugar molecules discover each other and return to the crystals.

Supersaturation and Precipitation

A limited quantity of sugar is dissolved in cold water, but greater temperatures enable the liquid to contain more sugar molecules. The hot liquid is a supersaturated solution. When the temperature is moderate, there is not enough space for the sugar molecules, so they return to a solid-state, translucent structure through a process called precipitation.

Growing Crystals

Crystals are growing and still not alive and they seem to produce order out of nothing. For these purposes, researchers have been excited for thousands of years. Crystals are prevalent and simple to produce, even if they require a little research to comprehend. Producing crystals and studying them is so intriguing that it may not seem like a work project at all.

CHAPTER 2
BEGINNING OF CRYSTAL HEALING

It's reasonable to say that as long as we've been a species, we've had an affinity with rocks and crystals. The use of talismans and amulets goes back to the origins of the human race, although we have no manner of understanding how the first of these artifacts were regarded or used. Many early parts were of organic origin. Beads sculpted from mammoth ivory were collected from a tomb in Sungir, Russia, 60,000 years ago (Upper Palaeolithic era), as well as modern beads produced from the shell and fossil shark teeth.

Crystal Healing has a lengthy, colorful past. Doctors, shamans, magicians, priests and healers utilized the energy of crystals in many ways.

Tribal societies handled rocks in ingenious ways, to predict the future, to interact with the ancestors and to cure illnesses.

Antique Egyptian civilizations used prolific healing crystals. Native American cultures have created comprehensive use of the protection and healing energy of many crystals. These and numerous other countries were in contact with the soil, the environment and their position as human beings in the natural world. Over the last five thousand years, mystics and magic have repeatedly told us that we belong to the world as mountains and trees. We disregard their wisdom in our peril.

The oldest amulets are Baltic amber, discovered 20,000 years ago. Amber beads were also discovered in Britain 10,000 years ago. The distance they traveled to Britain demonstrates the individuals of that moment their worth. Jet was also common and jet earrings, bracelets and necklaces were found in Palaeolithic tombs in Belgium and Switzerland. Malachite mines were proven to exist in Sinai as early as 4000 BC.

Amulets were prohibited by the Christian clerks in 355 AD, but gemstones continued to serve a significant part, with Saphir being the favorite gem for ecclesiastical seals in the 12th century. Marbodus, Bishop of Rennes in the 11th century, asserted that agate would make the wearer more pleasing, persuasive and for God's sake.

Historical References

The first historical references to the exploitation of crystals originate from the old Sumerians, who created magic formulas incorporating them. Ancient Egyptians used lapis lazuli, turquoise, carnelian, coral and transparent quartz in their jewelry. They sculpted tomb amulets of the same gems, too. Egyptians used rocks mainly to protect and preserve their health. Chrysolite (subsequently known as Topaz or Peridot) was known to help fighting night terror and drowning evil spirits. Egyptians made use of crystals in cosmetology as well. Galena (which is a lead metal) was crushed and was used as an eye shadow later labeled as "kohl". Another stone that has been used in a similar manner is malachite. Green rocks, in particular, were used to indicate the core of the dead and were included in the tombs. Green rocks were used contemporary in Ancient Mexico.

Ancient Greeks ascribed many characteristics to gemstones and lots of the denominations we now use have Greek origins. The term 'crystal' originates from the Greek 'ice' because it was thought that transparent quartz was water that had cooled so deeply, that it would always stay strong. The term amethyst implies 'not drunk' and was carried as remedy for intoxication and hangovers. Hematite was named after 'blood' because of the coloring it produces when it oxidizes. Hematite is iron ore and the ancient Greeks linked iron with the god of battle, Aries. Greek fighters would rub hematite all over their bodies, apparently to render themselves indestructible. Greek seamen also carry a range of amulets to protect them at sea.

Jade was extremely prized in ancient China and some Chinese characters represented jade crystals. Musical instruments in the shape of chimes were produced of jade and some 1000 years ago Chinese emperors were sometimes placed in jade armor. There are jade mask weddings in Mexico around the same period. Jade has been recognized as a healing rock for the kidneys in both China and South America. Around 250 years ago the indigenous population of New Zealand, known as Māori, wore jade pendants depicting ancestor spirits, which were handed down through the masculine line for many centuries. The tradition of fortunate green rocks remains to this day in areas of New Zealand.

Crystals in Religion

Crystals and gemstones were used in a way or another in all religions. They are referenced throughout the Bible, in the Koran and many other spiritual documents. The source of the birthstones is the breastplate of Aaron, or the "High Priest Breastplate," as stated in the Book of Exodus. The 4th of the seven Heavens in the Koran consists of a carbuncle (garnet). The Kalpa Tree, which constitutes an invitation to the gods in Hinduism, is said to have been built completely of precious stone and the Buddhist text of the 7th century mentions a diamond altar located close the Tree of Knowledge (the neem tree under which Siddhartha meditated). A thousand Kalpa Buddhas rested on this seat. The Kalpa Sutra, in Jainism, talks of Harinegamesi, the holy captain of the foot soldiers who captured 14 precious stones, cleansed them of their lower characteristics and kept only their best nature to help their changes.

There is also an old sacred lapidary text, the Ratnapariksha of Buddhatta. Some sources say it's Hindu, but it's most probable Buddhist. The period is unsure, but it's likely from the 6th century. Diamonds in this book are extremely regarded as the King of gemstones and are classified by caste. The Sanskrit term for diamond, vajra, is also the term for the Hindu goddess Indra and diamonds are often linked with thunder. The ruby was also greatly admired. It was an inextinguishable flame and it was intended to preserve the physical and mental health of the wearer. The treaty lists many other gemstones and their characteristics.

The Renaissance

In Europe, from the 11th century to the Renaissance, a variety of medical treatises extolled the merits of precious and semi-precious stones in the therapy of certain diseases. Typically, rocks have been used along with herbal antidotes. The creators were Hildegard von Binghen, Arnoldus Saxo and John Mandeville. References are also made to stones with specific power or safety characteristics. In 1232 Hubert de Burgh, prime justice of Henry III, was convicted of taking a gem from the king's treasury, which would render the wearer powerless and give it to Llewellyn, the King of Wales and Henry's foe. It was also thought that the gemstones were damaged by Adam's initial sins, that they might be populated by demons, or that if they were to be treated by a sinner, their qualities would disappear. Therefore, before carrying, they should be sanctified and consecrated. Today, there are reminiscences of this faith in the purification and programming of crystals before use in crystal healing.

The tradition of using precious stones in healing was still recognized during the Renaissance, but the inquiring minds of the era attempted to figure out how the method truly functioned and to offer it a more academic explanation.

The Beginning of Crystal Healing

In 1609 Anselmus de Boot, a court doctor of Rudolf II of Germany stateed that any virtue of a gemstone should be due to the existence of nice or bad angels. The good angels would bestow unique grace upon the gems, but the evil angels would tempt individuals to believe in the rock itself and not in the donations of God conferred upon it. He continues to mention some rocks as useful and to lay down the characteristics of others merely to superstition. Later in the same century, Thomas Nicols expressed in his 'Faithful Lapidary' that crystals, as lifeless objects, could not have had the impact believed in the past. Thus, in the Age of Enlightenment, the use of precious stones for healing and security started to drop out of favor in Europe.

A variety of exciting studies were performed in the beginning portion of the 19th century to show the impacts of rocks on people who thought themselves to be clairvoyant. In one instance, the topic asserted not only to feel physical and mental modifications when touched by multiple rocks but also to experience scents and flavors.

Crystal and Gemstone Meaning

In spite of no longer being in medicinal use, gemstones have persisted in having significance. Until lately, the jet was popularly carried by those in mourning and the grenade was often carried in wartime. There is a tradition in the local community here in the north of England: every woman descendant carries an antique moonstone necklace for her wedding, which has been in the community for centuries. It was only later that one family member realized that it was a sign of fertility.

Many indigenous societies have persisted in using gemstones for healing up till recent times, if not until today. The Zuni tribe in New Mexico is making fetishes of rock, representing animal spirits. They were ceremonially' fed' on powdered turquoise and ground maize. Beautiful inlaid fetishes are still produced for sale and are very collectible artifacts or carvings, although the spiritual practice that surrounds them is no longer very much in use. Other native American groups still retain sacred precious stones, particularly turquoise. Both Aborigines and Maoris have traditions concerning rocks and medicine or spiritual practice, some of which they share with the remainder of the globe, while some information remains personal within their societies.

It is essential not to forget that there are many instances of gemstones meaning comparable stuff to distinct societies, even though there has been no contact between these societies and no chance for a crossover. Jade was considered a remedy for kidney disorders by ancient

Chinese, as well as by the Aztec and Mayan civilizations. Turquoise used to be worn to attract strength and health and jaspers have almost always delivered stability and calmness.

A New Age Dawns

In the 1980s, with the emergence of New Age culture, the utilization of crystals and precious stones started to re-emerge as a technique of healing. Much of the practice has been taken from ancient traditions, with more data coming from testing and channeling. Katrina Rafael's books in the '80s and Melody and Michael Gienger's books in the '90s revived the use of stones.

Nowadays, a big amount of novels are accessible on the topic and crystals are frequently featured in magazines and newspaper articles. Crystal therapy crosses the limits of Christian and spiritual belief. Not perceived as a domain of alternative culture anymore, it is now seen as an appropriate and more popular complementary treatment and many schools are now offering it as a qualifying topic

CHAPTER 3
THE HEALING POWER OF CRYSTALS DO THEY WORK

Created over millennia, healing crystals bring life to the components of the Earth and the universe. Harnessing the energy of the Sun, Moon and oceans, the gemstones unite us with the Universe once we interact with them. Many individuals ask if the crystals have spiritual capabilities and while many tales depict the healing stones' impacts, it depends on your knowledge. Not every individual is capable of understanding crystal mending and it takes a deep level of consciousness to open your mind and soul to the practice, but once you start, the journey sprinkled with alluring, mysterious and particular crystals will thrill you.

People either believe in the healing characteristics of crystals, or they think it's as probable to operate as collecting rock from the floor and attempting to do magic.

The healing forces and methods to use them may seem like magic, but crystals have a scientifically sound history. While crystals are still seen as an option in healing, the explanation of why crystals do what they do truly sounds very logical. Undoubtedly, crystals oscillate at their frequency, just as body cells and your Chakras resonate with them. This implies that when we come into touch with crystals, these distinct frequencies fulfill and improve your physical, spiritual and mental equilibrium.

Crystals enclose the impressive ability to convert, absorb, augment and conduct energy.

We are energy. We are surrounded by energy in every form and crystals are the perfect conductors. The vibrations of the gemstones change based on the energy type that surrounds them, therefore every rock has a particular and distinct aftermath on each person. Originally, crystal therapy was used to readjust the energy centers known as Chakras and convert the features of the body, developing in this way a pure power range. It is also believed that the ability of crystals does not stop at the spiritual level, but the changes in the energy field also influence and heal the physical body.

What can crystals do for me?

Once you've started using crystals, an excellent method to harness their mending energy is to use healing stones to manifest your plans and what you dream of achieving in life. Regarding crystals, these otherworldly stones link us to the Earth since they are concrete, physical shapes with strong vibrations. This energy remains to link with you when you carry these intentional crystals near to your skin, or when you put them in your setting. With every idea and purpose, these crystals take up your distinctive vibrational energy and amplify the positive vibrations that you cultivate.

In this eerie world of energies, crystal frequency guides you on your trip because it enables you to find your purpose and reminds you of your attachment to Earth. The well believed out purpose is the starting point for healing crystals because the particular motives instilled in your regular habits of thought are also component of their energy.

Why do crystals work?

Clear Quartz existed since the beginning of time and ancient populations have used crystals as protective talismans, peace gifts and jewels. Today, glass represents 12% of the Earth surface and is used in almost every kind of industry, including timekeeping, electronics, data storage and more. If crystals interact through computer chips, then isn't it feasible that this vibrational energy could be converted in other forms? Furthermore, with their bond to the planet and their life-giving components, it is reasonable that crystals are widely healing, particularly since they left their mark in almost every precedent civilization.

Among the first bits of scientific proof concerning the strength of crystals is the research performed by IBM scientist Marcel Vogel. While observing crystals develop under a microscope, he realized that their shape had taken the form of anything he was talking about. He assumed that these shocks are the consequence of the continuous assembling and disassembling of bonds between molecules. He also evaluated the metaphysical strength of quartz crystal and demonstrated that stones could store ideas comparable to how recordings use magnetic energy to record noise.

Albert Einstein said that everything around us is energy and just like sound waves, your ideas match the sensations of everything that is manifested in your lives. Therefore, if you confide in the healing capacity of crystals, the positive energy of these rocks will deepen your faith.

Anytime, we can choose our ideas and, as we proceed on our trip, each day provides us with fresh difficulties and beautiful experiences. Healing crystals remind us to silence our thoughts while reconnecting to the mending energy of the Earth. Patience is a valuable experience to gather from crystals because just like the years it took for these gemstones to emerge and mold, learning to work with the power of crystals is also a long process. As you study, develop and grow, use them as a reminder to be thankful for the prosperity offered to you by Mother Nature and the enigmas of the Cosmos.

How do I choose a crystal?

Mending stones have been used since primordial times, so there is an abundance of information and experience passed down from generation to generation. Once you understand the principles of crystals, the best way of choosing the correct healing stones for your trip is by using your intuition. Specialists claim that the crystal is the one choosing you and not vice versa. Walk around the space and see the crystals that stand out from you. Whether it's the dazzling colors or the otherworldly shapes and patterns that draw you in, every crystal has a unique vibrational energy that works to clear blockages and ward off negative energy.

Finding the correct rock is like any wellness exercise. It needs patience while you're stilling your mind and realigning your mind/body equilibrium. Hold the rock in your palm and think softly about your aim. Notice if you feel emotions such as hot or cold, pulsation, or stillness and quietness. These are all indications that this specific gem is the perfect fit for your spirit.

It also helps to define a specific issue or challenge that you are presently experiencing. If you have difficulty focusing, Fluorite helps to clear up mental and emotional distress that can discourage concentration. To attract abundance, citrine enables you to express your thoughts by conducting the positive energy of the Sun. Carnelian is a strong crystal that allows creative juices to flow.

If you have trouble letting go of old ideas that no longer serve you, Black Turmaline is a strong gemstone for releasing unwanted models that may have transformed into poor practices. It might help you release all the bad vibes from your body and your environment. This stone also acts as a security talisman, which is crucial if you are an individual who can quickly pick up on other people's energy. Hematite is good for deflecting the harmful energies of others by helping you settle and resuscitating your essence using Earth's energy.

If you're looking for a more peaceful life, amethyst is one of the finest motivation crystals to comfort you and restore your equilibrium. Another gemstone that facilitates balancing your emotions is the moonstone, which provides you with assistance when you feel overly emotional or disconnected from your feelings. Rose quartz is also valuable for spiritual well-being because it closes and readjusts the heart Chakra, which amplifies self-esteem and the unreserved love of others.

Whether you're looking for crystals for aesthetic purposes or for attracting peace and tranquility to your lives, they're all working to raise your energy. If you feel comfortable holding the crystal in your palm or touching your skin, get prepared for the chance to rock with this old healing art.

What is an intention?

Reflections generate fluctuations throughout the universe, making setting intentions a strong instrument for attaining happiness and well-being. Having a definite objective gives us understanding into our ambitions, aspirations and principles. Besides, it empowers us to live in the present moment instead of being caught up in negative thinking habits. Intents are like magnets. They're attracting what makes them come true. Setting an intention is a strong instrument to achieve happiness. Creating an objective starts by setting goals that are aligned with your beliefs, ambitions and objectives.

> Decide what's important to you. Your principles are driving activities in your lives and you will need to acknowledge what counts to you if you wish to be fulfilled.

> Explore regions of your lives that need to be upgraded. Consider how you can enhance your relationship, career, personal lives, spirituality, wellness and society.

> Be specific about what you plan on doing, when you want to do it and why.

> Bring your intentions back to life. Some of the procedures explained in the next sections will invite you to write them down. Be sure to write them in the present tense as if they're going to happen now and only confirm what you want. It is important to write down your objective too, the aftermath of what you want to depict. Put the sensation in it!

I have my crystal. Now how do I behave?

One of the essential (and often ignored) elements to work with healing crystals is defining your intent or priority. Otherwise stated, you must assign a target to your crystal! Stones try to work for you, but you must guide them. During hard times, when you vibrate at low frequency, your thoughts can float out of the window. When you reconnect with your scheduled crystal, it will assist you in remembering your objectives and limitless possibilities.

The programming of your crystal is easy. Begin by cleaning up your crystal. You can choose your chosen wiping technique and what the most resonates with you. Immerse your crystal in the smoke of a burnt sage stick, Frankincense resin or Copal incense. Place your crystal under the sunlight or the full moon light for a couple of hours (I would suggest at least four). Bury it and let it recharge with Earth's energy. If it's a tiny crystal, you can position it on top of a translucent quartz crystal or a selenite one to purify it and clean up any stuck energy.

Next, keep your crystal in your fingers, near your eyes, take three profound breaths. Think about your faith, the earth and something that brings you happiness. This is going to bond you with your greatest vibration. Your highest vibration may be identified with a religious or sacred belief, a divine figure, or simply a power greater than you. Or it may be linked to a science connection—zero-point power. You're deciding what to call it. Then, while in this mindset of peace and light, pray for your crystal to be freed of any unwanted energy or prior programming.

5 simple ways to use crystals

If you're starting to use crystals, begin with these five strong and vital crystals of intent to foster equilibrium, harmony and peace of mind.

Clear Quartz and How to Use it

One of the most common crystals among beginners, transparent quartz additionally deepens your desire, making it the main element of a crystal collection. It's also the most flexible rock because it amplifies the motions of the rocks around it. Transparent quartz rods are usually used to clean and re-energize crystals. This is due to its strong purification impacts and the capacity to counteract adverse energy blockages.

Sit silently with a rock and think that its white light fills your flesh with beneficial energy. Contemplate your desire for the healing crystal and believe in the strength of its vibrations over the millennia harnessed from Earth.

Selenite and How to Use it

Selenite is another strong cleaning stone because it guarantees a favorable stream of vibrations between your body and other crystals in your collection, making it a perfect crystal for beginners.

Quickly extract adverse energy from your body and clear the aura around you by shifting selenite from your head to your toes. Repeat this purification routine for as long as you need to feel rejuvenated by positive vibrations. After that, you will enjoy a renewed feeling of equilibrium and the security of the white light that links you to the universe.

Shungite and How to Use it

One of the rarest rocks on Earth, Shungite includes antioxidants that give it powerful healing characteristics, including safety from dangerous substances that are detrimental to the body. Shungite is generally utilized to soothe anxiety and accelerate the detoxification process. This healing stone has strong physical impacts, so it's best to bring it gently.

Position a fragment of Shungite right next to your laptop, wi-fi hub, or other electronic devices in your house. We also suggest that you place a bit of Shungite on your cell phone to reduce the impacts of EMFs.

Amethyst and How to Use it

Known for its strong spiritual characteristics, the lovely amethyst is the perfect stone to decorate your house. This visually striking rock is also a great meditation tool because it enhances internal power and offers spiritual security.

As you focus on your purpose, position amethyst in your cabinet or dormitory to exhale calming energies and invitation in abundance. This stone also operates as a supplementary therapeutic instrument for yoga and meditation.

Citrine and How to Use it

Citrine harnesses the energy originated from the Sun. This rock is covered with light, making it ideal for placing it in the windowsill. Its regular infusions of natural light restore and regenerate its strong vibrations. Considered to be one of the strongest rocks for expression, citrine is essential for beginners, since it helps to transform your goal into reality. It also infuses a favorable perspective and stimulates the mind in such a way that you are encouraged to develop healthy practices and be always packed with optimism.

Position a fragment of citrine (we recommend a citrine point) close to your list of dream manifestations to make them come true much faster.

Not only are they brilliant eye candy, but these rocks also bring us back to Mother Earth and her incredible wealth. In the old art of crystal healing, gemstones rock when it gets to good vibrations!.

CHAPTER 4
THE SCIENCE BEHIND CRYSTALS

Is there any scientific proof that the crystals operate? It is an undisputed reality that quartz crystal has characteristics such as piezoelectricity, whereby its six ends alternate a favorable and negative charge under certain circumstances. And we understand that quartz can garner vast quantities of information and that crystals are used in everything from watches to computer chips to vehicles. Thanks to quantum physics, science now recognizes what the metaphysicists have been stating all along, that everything is energy, that energy can be transmuted and altered and that everything vibrates. It is also recognized that minerals don't need to be specifically ingested to be efficient and that healing is feasible throughout moment and space.

Historically, populations such as the Romans, the Ancient Egyptians, the Chinese, the Ancient Greeks, the Indians and the Ancient Japanese have used crystals to encourage relaxation, enlightenment and the appeal and satisfaction of all types of longing. The use of crystal dates back at least 6,000 years to the moment of the ancestral Sumerians of Mesopotamia. They are regarded to have metaphysical characteristics and some even assert psychic abilities periodically. So this contributes to the question, what's so unique about crystals?

All crystals (or, to be accurate, crystalline silica) is regarded to be one of the construction blocks of existence. They are produced of the two most common components on the planet–Silicon and Oxygen. The atoms bond together under stress, after which they form, extremely stably, into a three-dimensional model of repetition, providing the' crystal' its shape.

Silicon and oxygen together make up around 75% of the Earth surface. Silicon is also remarkable conductor of electricity and therefore crystals are of great use in the technology sector. These characteristics have rendered Crystalline Silica an indispensable element of the natural and technological worlds.

The glass–Quartz–is among the most secure glass buildings around and is therefore commonly used. It is widely used in transistors, in the universe of integrated circuits and is the cornerstone of all computer chips. It is utilized, as well, in all types of electronics, including phones, portable army radios and sophisticated electronic devices. In the sector of laser optics, this gem is used in the form of prisms and optical filters for timing devices. Certain crystals are also used for quartz watches and other similar equipments.

It seems that we are highly dependent on crystal technology in our daily life!

Of course, quartz is also an element of all types of land, dirt and sand. It is common in igneous, sedimentary and metamorphic stone formations. Certain microorganisms (radiolars) use a compound removed from water to create their buildings and shells. Quartz is also essential for craftsmanship in buildings. It is made of concrete and cement, as well as plastic, rubber and paint! Stone is between 70 and 90 percent quartz.

So, how do crystals function?

Quartz crystals have a very distinctive property called piezoelectricity. Mechanical stress is converted into electricity by a piezoelectric crystal. This implies that twisting or squeezing or compressing a crystal produces an electrical energy. The opposite is true as well; the electricity leads the crystal to flex, boost, or compress.

When a quartz crystal is ripped or smacked, the tension applied to it provokes an electrical charge. Once the electrical charge is transferred to the quartz, the crystal is distorted and when the voltage is withdrawn, the crystal generates an electrical field. It vibrates— sometimes 30,000 times a second! Considering that our bodies constantly produce energy, the relationship between us and the crystals is quite evident.

They also indicated that they have managed to collect vast amounts of information for more than a million years! Furthermore, the crystal was capable of thermal stability up to 1000.

Have a look at the technical spiel below if you dare.

"The prototype is made of a square of quartz two centimeters wide and two millimeters thick. It houses four layers of dots that are created with a second laser, which produces extremely short pulses of light. The dots represent information in binary form, a standard that should be comprehensible even in the distant future and can be read with a basic optical microscope. Because the layers are embedded, surface erosion would not affect them. "

–From the Scientific American Journal

This report implies that crystals (specifically quartz) can stock information through laser technology (which are effective wavelengths of energy). Moreover, it suggests that this mechanism works notably well with high-intensity fluctuations. This is especially beneficial in what concerns the absorption of other high-intensity electromagnetic waves like ionizing and non-ionizing radiation! Specific emission types (as sound, heat, sunlight) move at a lower speed and are not fully penetrating the body (non-ionizing), while other forms of radiation are faster-moving and extremely harmful (ionizing), which is the case of MRI scans and Gamma radiation. In these situations, the question is: do crystals have any properties that could be successfully used to lower the level of radiation?

The damaging effects of high intensity ionizing radiation appear to be at the core of our minds. The impact of radiation poisoning resulting from the bombing of Hiroshima and Nagasaki in 1945, for instance, can still be seen today. Nowadays, around 500 nuclear stations produce electricity around the Globe (only 10% of the total power). Following the Tsunami of 2004, a nuclear power station in Fukushima collapsed, resulting in almost one thousand tons of radioactive material discharged every day ever since into the Pacific Ocean! Subsequently, the devastating effects on underwater wildlife are alarming apparent. Could crystals maybe help to purify radiation poisoning within the oceans and absorb the high-intensity Gamma waves?

USING CRYSTALS AT NIGHT

Speaking of bedrooms, this is the perfect place for crystals, because they can assist us while we're sleeping. If we're in a dream-state, we can be more receptive to them, because our logical mind is switched off.

If you suffer from sleeping disorders, attempt putting a Selenite Tower on your bedside table, selenite is a fiber optic that captures the light and reflects it into the room. It produces a quiet room to assist with healthy sleep.

If you're keen in investigating your dreams, receiving texts through your dreams, or making a lucid dream, an attempt is putting a Labradorite rock under your pillow.

If you experience nightmares or dread during sleep, place Chrysoprase under the pillow or your bed.

You can also position four pieces of selenite, hematite or crystals in each corner of your room, creating a safety screen.

If I've had an emotional week, I'm going to sleep on rose quartz and it's not unusual to discover that I'm still carrying it when I wake up. Agates are also excellent crystals to keep while sleeping. Any rock that feels pleasant to hold on to it can assist you sleep easier.

Also for sleeping difficulties, attempt putting a grounding rock at the bottom of your bed like a Garnet, black tourmaline or a Jasper.

Finally, to help with detox during your sleep, attempt a bit of ocean jasper under your pillow or your bed. Make sure that it is rinsed and recharged with 20 minutes of sunlight every week or so.

These techniques are all cumulative. Luckily, there's not much you have to do, other than positioning the rocks, be receptive to them and let them get to work.

Remember that this is a vigorous exchange, which implies that you can take care of your rocks by maintaining them smooth, by loading them on your altar from moment to moment, or by burning a candle and putting them around it. The highest findings come when you remember to create room for appreciation every day.

CHAPTER 5
20 POWERFUL CRYSTALS AND THEIR HEALING PROPERTIES

Crystals are increasing in popularity these days, but these old minerals are also old spiritual healing instruments. There are numerous minerals generated in Mother Earth's pressurized womb that rise to the ground to become healing crystals that share their magic and knowledge with us.

Everything surrounding us is made of energy and stones, gems and crystals are no distinct. Each of them is produced up of small crystals in particular molecular structures that are continuously in movement, which also leads each rock and crystal to emit a distinctive vibration and characteristic energy field.

These unique energy vibrations interact with our energetic vibrations and can unequivocally affect us physically, spiritually and sentimentally.

Here Are 20 Powerful Healing Crystals and The Properties They Possess

These antique beauties are here to sustain us and will call us when we require their mending energy. Check out these

20 healing crystals and their characteristics to upgrade your spiritual level and even help you treating physical diseases you may suffer from. Which healing stones are speaking to you?

1. Selenite: The Master

This master mineral classified among the only healing crystals that need not be loaded and may be utilized to clean and recharge other crystals. It is the most common crystal, discovered in old evaporated salt lakes and oceans and can be discovered from Mexico to Brazil and beyond.

Metaphysical healing characteristics: Selenite is a conduit to the greatest point of consciousness and all that is infinite— spirit guides, the cosmos and curiosity. It brings the spiritual world to earth and it reminds us where we come from and where we are going.

Physical curative characteristics: Well-known for its master remedial properties, there's not much that selenite can't be used for. Meditating on the required result and bringing the stone with you can assist deliver excellent healing and inner peace.

2. Moonstone: The Stabilizer

Deeply connected to the female and the moon, the moonstone is the ideal rock to gently generate harmony within and reinforce intuition. It was a rock of divine figures in ancient India and it is considered sacred and royal.

Metaphysical healing characteristics: Moonstone has the ability to open you up to other realms and the Universe itself. It is useful to fight materialism and control the ego, as well.

Physical healing characteristics: Moonstone is utilized to help the pituitary and digestive systems, to fight against obesity, fluid retention, hormonal issues, menstrual issues.

3. Aventurine: The Stone of Opportunity

Recognized for amplifying luck, wealth and abundance, aventurine is a nice rock to bring with you if you're going to play in Las Vegas. Part of the quartz family, this rock draws good luck and helps the effective implementation of fresh possibilities.

Metaphysical healing characteristics: Correlated with the Heart Chakra, this gem can generate a feeling of overall well-being and mental calmness. It harmonizes the mental, physical and spiritual components and restores balance.

Physical healing characteristics: Aventurine supports the flow of the core, blood and energy and can assist speed up regeneration from injury, disease, or surgery.

4. Crystal Quartz: The Spirit Stone

Probably the most well-known gemstone, crystal quartz is viewed as a speck of light into the abstract world.

Metaphysical healing characteristics: this specific crystal includes the full spectrum of colors and can be easily utilized to augment wishes, rituals and manifestations from the nonphysical world to the physical one. Meditate on the glass and "program" the crystal with your wishes. Then you can wear or bring your crystal anywhere to amplify your energy and boost the manifestation of your wishes.

Physical healing characteristics: Crystal glass is a supreme healer and is believed to boost immunity and the circulatory systems and rise the flow of qi energy into the body.

5. Citrine: The Money Stone

The sort of quartz, the golden yellow color of this crystal, is connected with its association to cash, gold and prosperity.

Metaphysical healing characteristics: take this stone with you to the bank, to company conferences concerning finances, or put citrine on your table and look at it while you operate. Citrine can assist you gain riches and financial wealth and stabilization.

Physical healing characteristics: Citrine is considered to boost metabolism and support digestion and nausea. It is also possible to use it to reinforce nerve impulses, assisting the brain in burning more quickly and strongly.

6. Agate: Stone of Inner Stability

This diverse stone can be discovered in almost all colors with a big variety of striations. From clear transparent, stained and highly striped, agate personifies our inner nature.

Metaphysical healing characteristics: Agate increases self-awareness, stabilizes the aura (in all its colors), converts adverse energy and is a strong driving force of the spirit. Use this stone to cure frustration, mental disturbance and absence of self-worth.

 Physical healing characteristics: Known for enhancing mental function by enhancing the clarity of thought, agate is a fantastic rock that you can utilize before a significant exam, when composing, or when collecting ideas for significant discussion with someone you enjoy and want to interact effectively with.

7. Tourmaline: The Grounding Stone

Tourmaline, the preferred talisman of protection, is used as a psychic shield to base your energy and fight the introduction of adverse forces into your energy domain. Long used by sorcerers, shamans, witches and magicians, tourmaline can be discovered on every continent.

Metaphysical healing characteristics: Although tourmaline is a deep black, it can be used to remove adverse emotions, increase your vibration and bring you into the sun. Black absorbs light as it functions as a sponge for damaging or dark materials. It promotes you to stay radiant in dark moments.

Physical healing characteristics: use tourmaline to relieve pain in the joints and help to re-align the spine. It can also be used to reinforce the immune system, the heart and the adrenal cells–relaxing pressure and relaxing tension.

8. Rose Quartz: The Love Stone

This lovely purple quartz is connected with the core and expresses unconditional love for oneself, others and the planet.

Metaphysical healing characteristics: a marvelous stone that invites you to love, helps you to give love or attract a soulmate, rose quartz is all about the core. Wear or wear rose quartz to open up to discovering happiness if you're single and to deepen and nurture your love if you're in a partnership.

Physical healing characteristics: centered around the heart Chakra, this gemstone is useful for profound mental bonding and discharge and is known to enhance flow and reduced blood pressure. It is potentially helpful in relieving palpitations or missed beats and stress.

9. Turquoise: The Protection Stone

Believed to be the most antique gem known to humankind, turquoise has always been cherished by leaders, shamans, rulers, wizards and suchlike. Know as a sign of wisdom, turquoise is common in almost all old societies and has always been regarded as the rock of safety.

Metaphysical healing characteristics: Turquoise strengthens the intuition and meditation. It is also connected with the Throat Chakra, which promotes transparent communication, due to its black hue. Carry turquoise as a charm of safety and as a channel of old wisdom.

Physical healing characteristics: Assisting in mental issues, neck or ear pain and throat disfunctions, turquoise is very much linked with the psychic domain, making it an excellent rock to clear blockages and promote a good stream of energy throughout the body.

10. Fluorite: The Stone of Positivity

Perhaps this crystal is among the most underrated, but at the same time one of the strongest. This rock is regarded to pull adverse energy and small temperatures out of space or your body and to make room for the sun to shine in. Found in various color variants, fluorite is a magical crystal.

Metaphysical healing characteristics: used to protect the auric, increase your vibration, alchemize adverse energy and soothe a messy mind. Rainbow Fluorite is better known for stabilizing the mind and amplifying the psychic link and enhancing intuitive capabilities.

Physical healing characteristics: this vibrant rock can be used when learning to release your mind and sharpen your concentration. It is also useful to relieve body swelling, to dissipate cold diseases and to cure mucous membrane.

11. Lapis Lazuli: The Stone of Truth

This lovely, blue glass is among the most dynamic, old and sought-after crystals on earth. It has long been connected with royalty and luxury and its heavenly characteristics help the ones in the physical realm with wisdom and excellent judgment.

Metaphysical healing characteristics: Lapis Lazuli activates celestial upper Chakras and enables the Throat Chakra to communicate clearly and express one's thoughts easily. This fascinating stone encourages internal reflection and reality as it helps the exploration and depiction of the spirit realm.

Physical healing characteristics: use this strong stone to support and cure the neck, larynx and vocal cords. Because of its powerful links to the brain, it is thought to relieve Attention Deficit Disorder (ADD) by assisting the mind to concentrate and release useless thoughts.

12. Hematite: The Grounding Stone

This iron-rich rock is deeply grounded and linked to the earth. Mostly known as the "bloodstone" in ancient Greece because of the black hue of the iron material discovered in nature.

Metaphysical healing characteristics: Hematite directly affects the Root Chakra and possesses a deeply grounded energy that emphasizes our natural life and promotes us socially.

Physical healing characteristics: the iron discovered in hepatitis can assist us clean the blood, enhance circulation, handle uneven menstrual flow and promote a good body. It was also proven to be useful in liberating stress and anxiety and calming the nervous system.

13. Jade: The Dream Stone

This is another vibrant rock that can be discovered in a vast range of colors, worldwide. The region dictates the color and this stone is one of the most used. It has been celebrated across societies, centuries and millennia (and into contemporary times) for its physical and metaphysical healing characteristics, placing it among the most popular crystals known to man.

Metaphysical healing characteristics: jade reflects the nobleness of status and values. This rock is also linked to the core and enables us to acknowledge the reality, to communicate love (self and others) and to access the shamanic worlds in a dream state.

Physical healing characteristics: given the strong bond with the nucleus, Jade is useful for reducing toxins and purifying the body as a whole through the blood. It is also useful in relieving joint pain and speeding up the recovery process after surgeries.

14. Amethyst: The Manifestation Stone

Besides selenite and crystal quartz, it is one of the most encountered rocks in the New Age. Amethyst is present in a form or another everywhere on the globe. This lovely purple crystal is well recognized for many things, but the demonstration is the most important among the characteristics.

Metaphysical healing characteristics: connect with amethyst to your heart's wishes and life's intent and then express it in your life! This strong crystal is connected with the upper Chakras, assisting us in taking the etheric domain to the physical plane. This involves bringing to life our earthly dreams.

Physical healing characteristics: use amethyst to increase the sympathetic nervous system, equilibrium hormones, alleviate headaches, ease the stress in the throat and treat insomnia. Place the amethyst under your pillow at night to ensure that you can sleep profoundly and wake up relaxed, prepared to produce and communicate.

15. Kyanite: The Stone of Emotion

Kyanite helps the mind to build connections where none existed before, particularly in terms of mental growth and meditation. It does not collect adverse energy, so it does not need to be cleaned and can effectively be used to purify other rocks and rooms. The soothing blue-green tone is connected with the heavens and is therefore highly relaxing and nerve-friendly.

Metaphysical healing characteristics: Psychic skills can be improved by cyanite as it deepens meditation and connects pathways to the spirit realm. It might also help assisting those who are transitioning through death.

Physical healing characteristics: Cyanite is great to assist cure any pain in the neck and enhance communication. It is wonderful to relieve headaches, eye pain from looking at a laptop and neck strain.

16. Obsidian: The Mirror Stone

The jet-black rock is a mirror rock because of its capacity to improve the vision and the manner you see the universe and the situations. It's an extremely reflective surface and coherent coloring allow you to look profoundly inside to uncover your soul and the healing needed to raise your vibration.

Metaphysical healing properties: the use of the obsidian goes back to the Stone Age and its natural characteristics have been understood to allow the vision of other beings, of the soul itself and of places not available from the land, to achieve wisdom and understanding. Use this rock to disclose your shadows, faults and weaknesses in order to better comprehend yourself.

Physical healing characteristics: use obsidian to relieve emotional distress that has long been buried, overlooked, or even erased from memory. It is also a great remedy to relieve pressure and anxiety connected with mental trauma.

17. Blue Topaz: The Stone of Creativity

The light green color of the topaz represents the mind and our creative ability. It can assist boost the mind to learn more rapidly and to maintain data that can be used for years to come. It is also helpful in creating creativity and opening the mind to fresh thoughts.

Metaphysical healing qualities: since Topaz is a rock of the mind, it is good to connect with one's angels, spirit guides and close people whom you've lost. Use the topaz to expand your mind, open your soul and align yourself with the spirit realm.

Physical healing characteristics: Topaz has long been considered to help with mental illness, eye disease, dimness in vision and to recover loss of flavor.

18. Opal: The Eye Stone

This wonderful and colorful rock appears to be on fire with a rainbow spectrum of electrical colors as it moves in the sun. It's directly connected to the eye as it is so enjoyable to look at and linked with the pineal gland (Third Eye Chakra).

Opal inspires optimism, joy, gratitude and an overall feeling of well-being. There are over ten distinct kinds of opal, all from distinct areas of the globe with mildly distinct characteristics.

Metaphysical healing characteristics: Opal serves as an eyeglass of our auras, bringing the whole light spectrum into the body of spirit and energy. It can amplify the vibrant energy of the soul that is not frequently seen from other rocks. Use opal to awaken psychic and mystical characteristics and as a car for connecting with ancestral religious domains.

Physical healing characteristics: Opal can be used as an eye rock to assist promote eye wellness and enhance sight. It may also enhance memory and strengthen neurotransmitter disturbances.

19. Amazonite: Stone of Courage

Amazonite has the potential of calming the spirit and tranquilizing the soul with its gentle violet color. This rock empowers you to find out and communicate your internal reality with bravery and belief, without being overly sentimental.

Metaphysical healing characteristics: used to bring equilibrium and to purify the Chakras, amazonite can relieve the mental trauma stored in the body and assist avoid this trauma from occurring in a physical condition. It is also helpful to harmonize the connection between intellect and intuition for a good equilibrium that is grounded and enlightened.

Physical healing characteristics: typically used for overall well-being, amazonite is useful to the body as a whole. Use it especially to calm rashes, clear acne and deter wound infection.

20. Garnet: The Stone of Health and Creativity

This extremely grounding stone is present worldwide in different shades and designs. It is best regarded for its characteristics of encouraging wellness and the flow of creativity and attracting energy on Earth.

Spiritual healing characteristics: Garnet helps to eliminate inhibitions and taboos and enables the mind to believe freely and creatively. It encourages the individual to join the physical sphere and connects the channels of communication and creativity with the inner self to external speech.

Physical mending properties: well-known to boost metabolism, the granate is a fantastic rock to get stuff going in the body and, at the same time, to assist blood clot and prevent bleeding. Another great use could be in enhancing libido and sexual wishes.

Elevate Your Energy With Healing Crystals!

Healing crystals are magical, vibrant elements. There is a reason why humans have been using them for their healing characteristics from the dawn of history and they can assist you in living a more balanced and vibrant life when used correctly and with profound regard. They're nice to look at, but they're also highly strong.

Crystal culture has highly developed in the last century and it is increasingly essential to shop deliberately from vendors who supply crystals sustainably and with a deliberate aim not to over-harvesting these valuable items from Mother Earth..

CHAPTER 6
HOW TO CHOOSE A HEALING CRYSTAL THAT'S RIGHT FOR YOU

Crystals are beautiful–but they aren't just for show. Every crystal has unique properties and vibrations useful for different healing purposes.

Looking for a crystal can be overwhelming, particularly as a beginner. There are thousands of gemstones, each with its distinctive composition, power, color and usage.

In this section, we're going to speak about determining the correct type of crystal and then choose a particular rock that feels right for you.

Choosing the Right Type of Healing Crystal

Method #1: Let Your Intention Guide Your Choice

The simplest way to pick a healing crystal is to decide which region of your lives you want to enhance and then choose a crystal that resonates with that purpose.

Each crystal has distinctive characteristics that alter our energy field in many aspects. So, whether you're concerned in religious self-development, security, wellness, or overall well-being, there are various crystals that combine with that energy.

Method #2: Choose a Crystal That Resonates With a Chakra

Chakras are spiritual energy centers that are often described as spinning gears. They maintain us safe and balanced when they are accessible, but issues occur once they are clogged or unbalanced. Crystals can assist cure the blockages of the Chakra.

The main Chakras are aligned with the spine. They are connected to the nervous system and significant organs, along with our psychological, mental and spiritual being.

One color is assigned to each Chakra and every one of the seven main Chakras is linked to a specific rock. By defining the Chakra that you want to unblock or harmonize, you can determine the finest crystal to assist.

There is a list of the 7 main Chakras and the crystals associated with them:

Base Chakra – The color attributed to the Base Chakra is red, its main feature being grounding your energy. Known to be related with survival and protection this energy center is positioned at the root of your spinal cord. Among the stones linked with the Base Chakra we can find red jasper, bloodstone, black tourmaline and hematite.

Sacral Chakra – The Sacral Chakra is orange and helps the vital energy pass through your body. It's placed below your stomach button and is the nucleus of your artistic self, feelings, enjoyment and sexual organs. The crystals that vibe with the Sacral Chakra include amber, orange calcite and sunstone.

Solar Plexus – This lovely yellow Chakra is connected to your neural network. Its concentrate is on your power and self-confidence, assisting you in being your true self. The Sacral Chakra is situated just below your breastbone and resonates with citrine, rutilated quartz, pyrite and yellow jasper, among many others.

Heart Chakra – The beautiful green and pink Heart Chakra emanates love, compassion, unconditional love and forgiveness. It is placed at the midpoint of the chest and links the lesser physical Chakras to your greater mental Chakras. Stones that beautifully resonate with this Chakra are: emerald, rose quartz, green jade and green aventurine.

Throat Chakra – This sky-blue Chakra is the center of free-speech and communication and is situated at the lowest point of the neck. A higher importance of it comes from the fact that it is the first one amongst the spiritual Chakras. Turquoise, aquamarine, blue apatite or lapis lazuli are just some of the wonderful gems vibing with it.

Third Eye – This Chakra is a profound indigo color and the core of your intuition. Stimulating the Third Eye Chakra activates the pineal gland and enhances psychic abilities. It is heavily resonant with purple fluorite, amethyst, shungite and labradorite.

Crown Chakra – It is by far the most mystical Chakra and it is either purple/violet or white. It's your link to greater consciousness— divine purpose and destiny— and is situated at the top of your head. Few of the crystals connected with it are selenite, transparent crystal, amethyst and diamonds.

To choose a rock that is linked to a specific Chakra, it is useful to look at the personality, power and color of the crystal and how it resonates with you. There will be many crystals connected with each Chakra and some will merge multiple Chakras.

Method #3: Choose a Crystal That Resonates with Your Astrological Sign

There are twelve astrological or zodiac signs, one of which is linked to your birthdate. Choosing a crystal linked to this astrological sign is useful if you don't have a specific focus in mind.

Aries (March 21 – April 19) – People born under this Star sign are ambitious and good leaders. A choice of Ariens crystals includes meat, bloodstone, green jasper and citrine.

Taurus (April 20 – May 20) – Taureans are things that need to be predictable. They are faithful and trustworthy.

Connected crystals include jade, dioptase, malachite and amber.

Gemini (May 21 – June 20) – People born under this star sign can be changeable and they are excellent communicators, versatile and quick-witted. Some of the rocks that line up with Gemini are labradorite, agate, chrysoprase and tourmaline watermelon.

Cancer (June 21 – July 22) – Cancerians are caring, dedicated and sympathetic. They vibrate well with the power of the emerald, the pearl, the moonstone and the red jasper.

Leo (July 23 – August 22) – People born under Leo have strong self-esteem and are strong and vibrant. Onyx, carnelian, pyrite and purple topaz all re linked to the energy of Leo.

Virgo (August 23 – September 22) – This star sign is centered around assisting individuals and caring for the planet. Virgo's crystals include purple tourmaline, peridot, green jade and moss agate.

Libra (September 23 – October 22) – Librans are enjoyable, creative and smart. Sodalite, peridot, tourmaline and opal are all excellent crystals for this symbol of the star.

Scorpio (October 23 – November 21) – People born in the symbol of Scorpio are enthusiastic, responsive, charismatic and autonomous. Rocks as moonstone, rose quartz, topaz and beryl all resonate with the amazing energy of a Scorpio.

Sagittarius (November 22 – December 21)- The Sagittarians are sociable, hopeful and enjoy travelers. Stones corresponding with their vibe include sodalite, turquoise, tiger eye and topaz.

Capricorn (December 22 – January 19) – People in this star sign are ambitious, willing and self-disciplined. Some of the crystals that are linked to this astrological sign are tiger eye, hematite and malachite.

Aquarius (January 20 – February 18) – In all things, Aquarians like the truth and are very independent. Stones aligned with the Aquarian environment are granate, amethyst, opal and coral.

Pisces (February 19 – March 20) – The Pisceans placed their companions in front of them and they care to achieve their objectives and fulfill their aspirations. Pisces are connected to rocks as angelite, aquamarine, saphire and amethyst.

Conclusion

The choice of a crystal is interesting. It opens up a whole fresh universe of religious empowerment.

But it's not always simple or simple, particularly as a beginner.

The first stage is to determine your intent. What is your reasoning for choosing to use a crystal? What are you hoping to benefit from this?

Once you've chosen an idea, it's much easier to make a list of crystal kinds. You can begin looking for shops, internet stores, exhibitions and road sellers for a crystal that resonates with you.

It's often said that you don't choose a crystal, but the crystal selects you, so attempt not to get depressed or worried about having the ideal one. You may even be lucy enough to receive one as a present.

CHAPTER 7
COMPLETE CRYSTAL
FROM A TO Z

Letting crystals into your lives enables you to adopt old and mystical wisdom–but you also need the means to comprehend these rocks as they are today.

With our advice on your part, you will discover out all you need to learn about the healing crystals for spiritual growth.

Crystal Meanings

Abalone Shell

Alongside its marvelous ocean of colors, it is a protective rock, not least because it performs the same literal purpose in nature. At moments when your trust seems to be giving up, or you think uncomfortable, achieve your Abalone Shell for convenience and instruction.

This makes this stone popular in overcoming anxieties, but also in remaining true to oneself –particularly in issues of the core. If you sometimes discover that anxiety and self-sabotage are going to get in the manner of your interactions, this might be a rock for you.

Agate

Agate has been heralded for millennia as a rock of notable equilibrium and grounding energy. There is a good feeling of positivity within Agate, which implies that even the most skeptical of us can discover some hope for the future to let in the forces of this stone.

Agate functions because it links you to a wider view and allows you to see the pros and cons of any specified scenario, which makes it a nice rock for those of us wishing to join a fresh chapter in life–a fresh connection, a fresh career change and so on–securely and confidently.

Amazonite

There is an extensive amount of love and healing energy in the Amazon that can assist break the cycles of adverse ideas that you may be facing in your lives. In particularly pronounced instances, Amazonite can even assist in revealing and breaking through the karmic models of past incarnations and lifetimes.

Amazonite is often seen as a rock of courage–appropriate, perhaps, to be deemed Amazonian warriors! It can awaken you to your bravery and assist you in taking a position assertively, but compassionately, by breaking the illusions that keep you on a loop of errors, repeated all over again.

Amethyst

Always a guiding light for psychic professionals and a lovely crystal for use in jewelry, Amethyst is both common and strong.

It can awaken you to greater wisdom and link you advise from beyond the physical globe, but it is just as efficient as a rock for physical therapy. In addition to its capacity to ameliorate headaches and joint pain, Amethyst also carries a feeling of peace.

Because of this, it's a nice crystal to decrease mental pressure and to stop your brain from concentrating on the same thoughts of uneasiness repeatedly, disturbing sleep and concentration.

Apatite

Ambition and a feeling of life-enthusiasm are all enhanced when the emotions of Apatite are allowed into yourself. This stone is colored in a wonderful shade that enhances the clarity of your mind. It can be fascinating to look at.

Apatite is regarded as a nice rock for creative thinking, meaning that it is not only useful for those who operate in the press and the arts but also that it unlocks fresh, innovative ideas for researchers and business-minded individuals. This is a flexible rock, with plenty to give to all fields of existence.

Apophyllite

With its frosty white and cool blue hues, Apophyllite is a wonderful rock to calm an overactive mind. It can also assist avoid over-energized poor habits, such as nervous twitches and tics.

Apophyllite, though, is a rock that is as much about avoidance as it is about a remedy. It operates by putting to light the root causes of certain activities and bad habits of lives. It may not be necessarily a pleasant method, but it is essential for spiritual growth and fresh stages of soul development. This stone, too, helps to alleviate the strain of these changes.

Aquamarine

As the name suggests, Aquamarine is a rock that is extremely bound to water and its beauty, nutritious characteristics. You may well think that the core of existence itself awaits you in this rock, so powerful that it's cleansing powers can often be.

But this is also a rock about the tides of transition in life. When you have difficulty getting away from challenging circumstances and interactions, Aquamarine connects you to your internal power. It can also assist you in positioning yourself with other individuals on the same trip.

Aventurine

Aventurine is a stone that is tightly linked to the Heart Chakra and that's where some ancient sayings about pursuing one's soul are born. Harmonizing with the adventurous vibrating nature of this crystal, these ideas encourage you to follow your heart with boldness!

There is a sense of playful risk involved with Aventurine. Many have named it the Gambler's Stone, thinking that it links you with nice luck and fortunate spots. While luck is perceived differently by every individual, it hardly hurts a little opportunity to come one way!

Azurite

Azurite is often referred to as the Stone of the Heavens, making it a common option for those who seek to adopt divine advice and ties to the angelic domain. This precious stone helps to open one's mind to what a solely pragmatic mind would find impossible.

It's a rock of faith and belief in a divine figure. However, it also encourages self-confidence with just as much power and it can assist you to keep up with vibrant thoughts as and when they hit, proud of your achievement. This crystal also helps to remove stress and concern.

Black Tourmaline

Same as many stones that share its density and color, Black Tourmaline is a guardian stone that protects you from adverse energy.

The crystal has, therefore, become particularly famous with individuals who are naturally empathic, or otherwise capable of absorbing the feelings and energy of others. Black Tourmaline is a powerful barricade to protect you from turmoil or emotional blackmail. It's a true supporter of trust!

However, the more you learn to operate with its energy, the more the crystal becomes useful to safeguard areas and other individuals.

Bloodstone

Despite its possibly provocative title, Bloodstone is very much in your hand, as you'll find out if you begin operating on crystal healing with it. It might help to relieve all sorts of body pain and injuries, or to elevate the effective circulation of blood and through the energy centers of your spiritual body.

Bloodstone is in direct connection to the root Chakra, which is the one that holds you most in physical truth. This is a rock to enjoy the moment, then and experience the pleasures of life. Nevertheless, when utilized in meditation, it becomes a precious anchoring stone that keeps you from going too far into the ethereal domain.

Blue Lace Agate

This is a calming and serene crystal, even if one looks at its colors alone. This stone has a mystical appearance and a lot of depth in the manner light performs even the easiest part of it.

It is linked to your capacity to shape and articulate your thoughts. If you often discover yourself overthinking and criticizing yourself for not taking up against unfair situations declining favors that you ask you to understand are too far-reaching, this crystal can assist you.

It's going to inspire firm but compassionate words that get your point across and it's going to help you see that most people making such requests don't try to be unkind to you.

Bronzite

While the majority of these stones specialize in one specific Chakras, Bronzite is one of the more unique crystals, able to bond with all of your Chakras. It puts them into balance and helps you figure out which parts of yourself most need healing and attention.

Bronzite, however, is a rock that also has many protective characteristics. It enables you to acknowledge when individuals are attempting to take the wool over your eyes and it is also great in triggering the greater components of your immune system. The feared office bug unexpectedly appearing out of nowhere could impact you less frequently!

Carnelian

The vibrant orange of Carnelian might sound like the warmth of sunset, but this is one rock that leaves you all but weary. There is a powerful undercurrent of vitality in this rock that perks you and electrifies your mind with thoughts and aspirations.

Carnelian is also linked to your sacred Chakra, where many pleasures of life are experienced and handled. If your "joie de vivre" is lower than the usual, Carnelian is the stone you need to reinvigorate your lust for life and you're chomping to the point of success.

Celestite

Exploring beyond our physical bodies becomes even easier when Celestite is around us. This rock seems to many to be a direct line to the sky themselves and in the same way, under the forces of this stone, you can relate much more simply to your higher self.

Celestite is the precious stone that is forevermore attracted to those who actively lead a spiritualistic existence, seeking reality, helping the poor, exercising altruism and meditating regularly. However, it also enables those who are just going out on their soul to discover their spiritual legs without feeling daunted.

Chrysocolla

As far as conversion is concerned, it is generally either our goal or the occurrences of existence that force us to alter–sometimes with or without our permission! But regarding Chrysocolla, with divine guidance, you will find that you are able to stimulate constructive change in your life.

This gemstone, with its wealthy earth colors also establishes a wonderful connection with nature. Same as seasons follow their cycle, you will be able to understand the rhythm of your life–and feel empowered to either cherish or interrupt the cycles according to your needs.

Chrysoprase

Although a plain pale green rock may appear, at first sight, Chrysoprase has many concealed depths. In reality, it could be said that this is a perfect stone for digging deeper into your soul too.

This is a rock of reality and enlightenment, which means that besides seeing the lies of others, you will also prevent involving yourself in certain fields of existence. By virtue of the powerful matters of compassion and love that dissipate the energies of this crystal, it is wonderful for mending and conquering traumas.

Citrine

Vibrant in color and also in its energies, Citrine is a gemstone that cannot assist but stimulate positivity and determination. It binds to your solar plexus Chakra, which is where most of the power transfer between individuals truly takes place, as well as some intuitive perspectives–or' good emotions,' as we often call them.

But in addition to enhancing these components of ourselves, Citrine also encourages the concept of development, including personal growth, the progress of a partnership, the evolution of an economic surplus–whatever you concentrate your forces towards.

Citrine boosts your trust appropriately, too, so if you've been feeling on your back foot recently, switch to this crystal to assist you in getting back on track and getting prepared to talk to your item.

Clear Quartz

Look no further than the very title of this crystal to comprehend its hidden healing strength. In other words, Clear Quartz operates by adding simplicity to all around you, allowing you to see the reality of stuff. Luckily, when these truths are a bit hideous or difficult to manage, this crystal also has relaxing energies that stop you from getting too harmed.

Clear Quartz is capable of healing the body and mind with equivalent smoothness, but its specialty is perception–both physical and mental. If you've been suffering from brain fog, or if you've had a confused mind owing to the stress you've experienced, this stone can make things straight for you, providing you a wider view on what to do.

Dalmatian Jasper

Sweet and speckled, Dalmatian Jasper is a precious stone of pure playful energy. If you've somehow forgotten the little joys of life, or you don't seem to have fun in anything you do, this crystal can reinforce your more frantic side.

This glass also enables you to meet the difficulties that come into your lives with a sense of humor—even the wisest of spiritualists understand how strong such a thing can be in the play of life! Dalmatian Jasper gives you a spring in your step and a joy in your heart, but don't worry—it won't leave you spaced out, either.

Dumortierite

Nowadays, everything seems to have to be instant and it can cause even the best of us to have some irrational aspirations. Good things come to those who wait and Dumortierite understands it. Use this crystal to help you see the larger voyage we're all going on and not to sweat the little things.

But in addition to patience, this crystal also encourages fulfillment and the capacity to react deftly to unpredictable modifications in lives. This rock will also reveal the interactions around you that are pulling you down and any toxic factors in your lives will discover their real colors revealed for all to see.

Fluorite

The vivid colors of Fluorite create it a famous stone in its own right, but it is the soothing characteristics of this rock that have made it so well-known. In an age characterized by stress and anxiety disorders, this crystal is a welcome, relaxing relief for the spirit.

Fluorite is a common meditation aid, not least because the state of extreme calm and quietness of mind is so essential for joining the meditative state. However, it may also be helpful if you have trouble sleeping. Just place it under your pillow.

Fuchsite

The majority of healers see Fuchsite as a rock of hard love. While it is invaluable to pierce through illusions, dispel bad karmic models and otherwise break up anything that holds you away, it does this with an energy that is very direct and touching.

However, the data and knowledge that this stone can assist you in relating to are far more important than any mollycoddling–and by being aware of the power of this stone, you will be able to recognize lies and deceit long before they have the opportunity to do any damage.

Garnet

Garnet is popular for being a wealthy purple color and in the same way, this crystal can arouse a warm red enthusiasm. But it's not just about love and it's about enthusiasm for anything else in life that you enjoy–art, practice, leisure, or hobbies.

Garnet helps to encourage you to take advantage of every day and it can assist to cure you physically so that you have the strength and energy to do just that. If you've felt a little caught in a rut, a gemstone can motivate you to stir stuff up in a favorable manner.

Goldstone

It makes sense, of course, that individuals who seek their luck often depend on the energies of Goldstone. It attracts abundance as well as curiosity and it also has a sense of excellent luck. With Goldstone in your hands, you can't assist but feel like there's a large windfall around the corner!

It is a stone of optimism that we could all be confronted with in today's globe of adverse media bias and ever-increasing difficulties before us as a community. Goldstone helps you to find the inner spark of brilliance within you and also gives you the ability to become a force, attracting positive changes around you.

Green Calcite

If you are interested in getting back into harmony with nature, or if you're attempting to discover methods to escape the folly of big city life, Green Calcite can only demonstrate a ticket. It's got this magical value of creating life easy just a little–just enough to take some precious time for you to sit on the beach or stroll through the park.

Green Calcite reminds us all that rest are as essential as curiosity and achievement when it relates to life's progress. Meditation with this crystal also awakens you to the patterns that direct a lot of lives and through this method you can comprehend your cyclical nature.

Hematite

The shiny shine of Hematite may well help to enhance your steely strength, but it also reinforces your physical body. This implies that it allows you to conquer sickness and injury, but it also provides you higher resilience to disease and fatigue.

Hematite focuses the mind and the heart of what is real, tangible, physical and attainable. If you find your head too often in the clouds, or even if your dreams at night are so intense that you are shocked to wake up, this rock can offer you precious grounding energy.

Jade

Crystals that are wealthy in culture and folklore are not much better recognized than Jade. Its link to the Aztecs and ancient China is well known and mythology has been around this rock for thousands of years.

Jade's reputation for safety, inspiration, motivation and healing is just as precise today. This is a lovely, flexible and extremely sought-after rock and its energy and beauty only seem to grow with era.

Jade provides wisdom and abundance to those ready to operate with his talents and he can open your eyes to the inherent duality of existence.

K2 Stone

Named for the pinnacle of the Himalayas, K2 Stone is equally eager to assist you rise to fresh heights. It is, in reality, a mixture of rocks mingled together and its colors are like a vivid summer sky.

This rock is said to amplify one's capacity to withstand the hard circumstances of existence. Sometimes, no matter how many crystals we may use, we will find ourselves unable to change the bad situation the moment we need it. Instead, we need to go through the process to its completion before we can finish it.

Similarly, in terms of physical therapy and wellness, this crystal demonstrates to us that some medical circumstances need to be taught to live with.

Kambaba Jasper

There is an almost animalistic value to Kambaba Jasper, particularly in its appearance. This precious stone talks to the more primordial components of ourselves and promotes us to understand that some items are just a component of human nature.

Of course, there is still every reason to try enlightenment and to go beyond ourselves in spite of that. But Kambaba Jasper will assist you in maintaining your power and perseverance throughout these procedures, as well as reminding you to take it easy on yourself if things go wrong. After all, you're only human!

Labradorite

This stone looks like a mix of all magical and ethereal colors that you could imagine swirling into forms within a piece of it. The many colors of this stone, particularly its blues and greens, demonstrate how it gives harmony to various Chakras, such as the neck and heart Chakras.

Labradorite amplifies your spiritual vibrations and connections. This implies that using it in meditations will often give you a much livelier experience and a piece of this rock under your pillow inspires colorful, insightful dreams at night.

Lapis Lazuli

The elevated vibrations of Lapis Lazuli create it a crystal that appeals to anyone who wants to fast track their intellectual development. Of course, there are no true shortcuts to enlightenment, but there are methods to increase your receptivity to divine advice and this stone is one such way.

This crystal encourages a straightforward mind, frankness and honesty in your communication. It enables you to link greater concepts and views with more simple rules of life and to see your physical and spiritual self as two halves of the same whole.

Leopard-Skin Jasper

The places and places that create the unique colors and markings of this gem assist in showing that we all have our styles and features. This stone and its vibrations help you to see that there is no shame in being who you are.

But, of course, doing so implies lots of mending and development–so, fortunately, this stone can help with that, too. It links the multiple points within you that will assist you break the bonds that hold you away from being your greatest self. But it also provides you the compassion you need to excuse yourself and all the others who might have wronged you along the manner.

Lepidolite

Lepidolite is correlated with development, but it also reminds us that advancement requires time. It's also sometimes awkward or depends on the old or obsolete being demolished or left behind.

The larger image is put into perspective when you operate with the healing fluids of Lepidolite. It will give you the power to take a step back and observe the course of life from afar and further, to take heart in the knowledge that any discomfort that you may encounter in your way today is only temporary.

Lepidolite enables you with all elements of conversion, including physical development, which means it's a nice dietary help or a fresh perspective.

Malachite

One of the most popular green crystals, Malachite is a rock that is deeply attached to the heart Chakra. This detail implies that it is a strong partner for any trips of the core that you may be creating, even if you're searching for responses in your love lives.

Malachite is also used energy to tap if you're recovering from heartbreak, or, in other words it is very effective in unlocking an obstructed Heart Chakra. It can also assist with chest pain, pulmonary problems and even circulation throughout the body.

Mookaite

This crystal is deeply attached to all that is physical and concrete. This implies that it can assist you in your manner to material success, but it also implies that it has grounding forces that stop you from becoming so stuck in daydreams that you never take action.

Action is indeed the name of the match for Mookaite and the biggest benefits of this rock come to those who use their talents to create great strides in life or travel. If you are interested in broadening your horizons, discover a fresh language, or discover a fresh nation, Mookaite is the rock to choose from.

Moonstone

A smooth appearance and heavenly texture made Moonstone a point of interest for those who seek to extend their dreams beyond what is feasible on this globe alone. In tarot and astrology, the moon is associated with secret feelings and hidden intentions, though not necessarily cruel ones—and the same is often true of this crystal.

Moonstone is particularly useful at soothing rifts in romance and at the same time promoting fresh enthusiasts to open their hearts to each other. Moonstone can encourage calmness and serenity to a worried pair and it is also able to illuminate any faults that prevent romance from working out.

Obsidian

Thanks to its black color and its overall lust, Obsidian is very evocative and mysterious. Anyhow, same as the majority of black crystals, the main forces at job in this rock are defensive ones.

If you often feel bowled over by the powerful characters of others, or otherwise find it difficult to surpass the lukewarm individuals, this stone will keep you safe and it can also assist you to talk your mind. At the same time, Obsidian is a rock of self-reflection and it will persuade you to analize and work on eventual flaws that you might otherwise not discover.

Ocean Jasper

Life may sometimes feel as unknowable as the ocean, but Ocean Jasper reminds us that we can at least navigate the waves of life appropriately. This stone will remind you how important is to relax and acknowledge that many of life's greatest journeys are the unplanned ones, those that might guide you to unknown locations .

Keep it close by when you feel enclosed. This crystal is going to help you find the surface and float whenever you feel drowned by your circumstances.

Onyx

Deep and mysterious, Onyx is a protective stone like many darker crystals. It is also a rock capable of awakening your internal trust and it can assist you to discover a healthier equilibrium of humility and self-esteem.

If you think that individuals have been wandering all over you or exploiting your generosity for too long, Onyx might be able to support you to stand firm. If you've been captured in what feels like an unlikely choice, too, then Onyx can assist you improve your decision-making skills.

Orange Calcite

The summer sunshine feeling of this stone helps boosting your confidence, as well as giving you the understanding you need into the excellent possibilities that come your way. It often requires bravery to reach out to fresh possibilities as they arise and this crystal will assist you do just that.

However, if you feel haunted by the events of your past, or otherwise you cannot let go of ancient pain, this crystal can help you cure these religious injuries, although it can also break your connections with them. It'll feel like a fresh lease of existence, ensuring you can contribute to the job of your soul.

Peridot

Peridot is a rock that emanates light and with it a feeling of positivity and abundance. This is a rock of abundance and it can also assist in transforming your mind around if you often discover yourself caught in a kind of narrow-mindedness.

Peridot has healing and inspirational characteristics that render it very famous among innovative intellectuals, but also a practical aspect that implies that those searching for strong alternatives can adapt its strategy. This rock operates tightly with your heart Chakra and helps you discover an equilibrium between doing things for others and taking care of yourself in the most efficient manner feasible.

Picture Jasper

There's a wealthy unrefined characteristic of Picture Jasper that encourages grounding energy and general gratitude for not rushing things when you don't need to. This might help you to stay steadfast and unshakeable in the pursuit of your objectives.

It's nice to be somehow shy. Otherwise, we can be so readily dissuaded from what we set out to do. This gem keeps you on your way and helps you to stay committed to your purpose.

It's also a crystal that attracts abundance to you, meaning it's common with those looking to increase their funds or their excellent luck in other parts of the material world.

Pyrite

You probably already know that Pyrite is also named Fool's Gold, but don't let your relative absence of currency quality fool you! In reality, it is a great partner in assisting you discover your luck and to adopt the thoughts you need for it.

Pyrite also encourages self-reflection though and by taking your time to analyze and know this stone, you will discover new features that aren't necessarily serving your higher cause. If you are looking to end bad habits or overcome what is holding you back, Pyrite is your friend.

Red Jasper

The wealthy color of this rock is mainly connected with the root Chakra–the very Chakra that connects each one of us to the physical globe. However, at a more affordable stage, this crystal will call your attention on self-care.

Red Jasper and his energies are naturally nurturing and they promote you to slacken if things go wrong or if you create lapses in judgment. Likewise, if you've been ill, the energies of this rock can assist you recover quicker.

Rhodochrosite

The cute cotton candy color of Rhodochrosite is a nice measure of how this crystal is perceived as a treat. While it's inexpensive enough, it's a rock to be nice to ourselves and to remember that we deserve affection.

If you've been putting your needs on hold for a while and now you don't know how to make yourself comfortable again, that crystal can assist you. It will remind you of the simple things you like and give you the means to connect with them and make yourself a little more upbeat and ready to face the challenges of life.

Rhodonite

Looking at a lengthy match is what Rhodonite is helping to encourage. This crystal has the potential of giving you a perspective into the habits of life and enabling you to acknowledge that sometimes you must plant plants well ahead of their harvest to take the best advantage of them.

It can direct you intuitively when creating savings or preparing a professional route and it can also assist you in choosing a long-term mate with whom you can travel a distance. However, when unforeseen occurrences happen, this crystal also enables you not to give up stuff so readily and remain the course.

Rhyolite

This is a crystal that allows you to see current conditions from a fresh view. This isn't always simple, but this rock can assist create it occur.

Likewise, if you feel like your existence became flat and monotonous, you can see it as though it had a new impact on this stone's energy.

Rhyolite is characterized by optimism, but it does not encourage any doubts in search of it. If you want a perfect equilibrium between your pragmatic self and the more optimistic one, Rhyolite is a nice crystal to look at.

Rose Quartz

Unconditional love understands no bounds, as Rose Quartz and her energies understand all too well. It is, by definition a symbol of romance. Furthermore, it symbolizes love of the family, of one's profession, or even of the force of life itself. Works like a charm in case you've been feeling apathetic lately!

This rock also promotes feelings that go hand in hand with love, such as compassion and forgiveness. If you're interested in curing distinctions of view or cracks in otherwise near friendships, this crystal is recommended.

Rutilated Quartz

Rutilated Quartz is appreciated by many faith healers and spiritually minded crystal enthusiasts because of how adverse substances can be so efficiently filtered out of your lives. If you find yourself defeated by pessimism in everything around you, this crystal can restore that view to a more balanced one.

It can also assist you to clean up your negativity, too. It can cleanse your soul and mind from any anger you have, even if it occurs to be subconscious. Many of these adverse feelings can slow down your religious development, making this stone a precious ally.

Selenite

The nature of life and warmth makes Selenite an important crystal for anyone who wants to see the spiritual truth in ##s. It is known for helping to open your third eye Chakra and, because of that, it can direct you to some intriguing spiritual ideas.

It's a crystal of purification, both yourself and your environment. Many individuals look to position Selenite in their home or office to maintain adverse feelings and small vibrational energies at bay. By maintaining yourself bright and airy, you are often prepared to be your greatest self.

Serpentine

Serpentine is a rock that operates with the lesser Chakras and, as such, can assist in easing any concern you have with the physical globe–or with physical pleasure.

If you are so anchored in the physical world that your greater and spiritual self is completely out of equilibrium, this crystal may even be a bit of a scale. And, of course, its color helps to awaken you to the curing power of nature, as well as how you can take greater care of yourself.

Serpentine is a crystal that helps to bring wealth in all its types, making it a good luck charm for many individuals.

Shungite

Shungite is a dark stone, but also one that has been ascribed to innumerable healing opportunities. Among the most valuable of these is the detoxifying characteristics of crystal, which means that bad lifestyle decisions can be countered a little by this rock.

Without doubt, the crystal also enables you to have self-discipline to adhere to a healthier lifestyle. There is an aspect of Shungite purity that can assist you acknowledge how to maintain stuff easy when you need to.

Smoky Quartz

If you feel that your advancement in life has been overshadowed by adverse emotions, Smoky Quartz can assist to cure that, as well as conquer the pain.

Smoky Quartz is a precious stone that allows you to reconnect to the wonders of being alive. Every day starts to feel like a fresh chance under this energy and the positive vibrations that you will receive from this crystal will help you see the possibilities in front of you.

Smoky Quartz enables you to discover mental equilibrium and it also takes you into higher balance with those around you–perfect if you've been overwhelmed by someone's late conduct.

Sodalite

Sodalite is, in many ways, one of the great equalizers of the world of crystal. If you feel so negative that you can't motivate yourself to create any adjustments to your lives– or so filled with favorable feelings that your feet never touch the surface–Sodalite puts everything into balance.

At the same time, Sodalite is also heavily related to spiritual vibrations and to align itself with your most deep intuitive ideas. Sodalite has grown into a very famous meditation rock because of this and that implies that you will be prepared to encounter fresh perspectives through these trips into yourself.

Sunstone

Few crystals can fuel up your artistic part like Sunstone. More than that, this crystal can enhance your ideas with grounded thinking, which means that once you start seeing new opportunities and perspectives in life, you won't feel stunned about how to follow them.

Better yet, this is an outstanding rock for trust. Have you ever had a wonderful concept to give it up because everyone seemed to speak it down? Sunstone is going to encourage you to stick a little more to those bright ideas. You never understand what awe-inspiring strides you could make if you permit yourself to thrive like this!

Tiger's Eye

Befitting the name, count on this stone to give you the guidance you need during times that require courage. It awakens a fearless part of you, in a way that isn't superficial.

That's because self-esteem and a deeper insight into yourself –your strengths and your weaknesses –is the kind of energy that Tiger's Eye offers. Confidence comes from just these kinds of insights and so it's only natural you'll be braver for coming to terms with these sides of yourself.

Tourmalinated Quartz

This distinctive stone has strands and streaks of Tourmaline in the body of the Quartz and it likewise combines clarity and strength in one handy package. It has the capacity of magnifying our natural energy, to activate our best-selves, at the same time allowing introspections, self-reflection and meditation on our own needs and dreams.

Through these discoveries, you will feel emboldened in following your life path with renewed passion. This type of Quartz motivates individuals on being self-sufficient and choosing wisely when in need of support.

Tree Agate

Just as how great things can come from small beginnings, Tree Agate can help you to better manage your ideas, visions and plans now, so that they can endure the test of time in the long term.

This stone favors mending and contemplation. It will offer you a better perspective on any concerns that you might encounter in your love life and it will help you achieve a deeper understanding of natural cures and will bring you closer to the spiritual realm, far from the chaos of the city.

Turquoise

Turquoise is a crystal that has remarkable ties to the throat Chakra. It is known for being used in earlier times as a healer against head colds, flu, allergic reactions and sore throats.

But on a more spiritual level, the strong attachment to the throat Chakra also makes this gemstone great at improving your communication skills. If you have experienced feelings of alienation, if you've felt like being cut off your friends group or tongue-tied when trying to connect to your prospective new partner, Turquoise can be a crystal to rely on.

As you can see, crystals are countless, they come in different shapes and the most important thing by far, humans have discovered infinite ways of using them. Many of these precious stones have reminiscent names, inherited over the ages, like "Petrified Wood" or "Apache Tears", but getting behind the mythology of crystals is simple once you have a clear starting point.

We can affirm, without any doubt, that our study provides all the needed information one might need in order to conduct a research on crystals and how these precious stones ensure healing, growth and development of body, mind and soul. These in-depth articles will guide you in your journey of choosing the crystal that best fits you, making sure it will improve many aspects of your life as well as helping you develop your intuition and extrasensory qualities.

CHAPTER 8
HEALING CRYSTALS:
10 MOST EFFECTIVE
HEALING STONES

Have you ever tried using healing crystals before? You might want to attempt using them, but you don't know where to start? Crystal Healing is used to cure individuals and their energy systems by putting crystals on and around the body, which can assist in extracting any adverse energy.

There are several different kinds of crystals that are used for distinct purposes. I'm supposed to speak about the top ten healing crystals and their significance. But first, let's talk about what healing crystals are and what they can do.

How Does Crystal Healing Work?

Research in the framework of the atom over the last few hundred years has disclosed that everything in our entire universe is composed of energy. Even strong items, like a piece of furniture or hair on your head, are only waves of energy at the most basic level. It may not look like your eye, but the healing crystals and cells in your body are created from the same energy.

Scientists have already discovered how to use the energy contained in crystals for all types of tasks, such as maintaining time using tiny quartz crystals on your watch or producing electronic components on your laptop and smartphone. Whether or not you understand it, the vigorous characteristics of these precious stones and rocks are commonly used in our contemporary technology.

We even use crystals in our medicines. Many pharmaceuticals are produced by grinding up minerals that shape inside healing crystals. Although our culture has several applications for the active characteristics of crystals, we have forgotten to standardize their use in natural healing.

Healing crystals work in the same way magnets do- attracting or projecting energy. When you position a crystal on a certain area of your body, your energy vibrates, pulses, moves and changes following the characteristics and energy of the crystal.

If you're looking to cure some part of your mind, body, or spirit, there are three main methods that healing crystals can turn your energy and fix the imbalance:

Clearing–Crystals are capable of absorbing and removing certain kinds of electricity from your body. Like a magnet can pick up small bits of metal shavings, a healing crystal can absorb adverse energy from your body.

Energizing–Healing plants and rocks can also drive power into your body, mind, or spirit through causing resonant vibrations. It is a very similar process to how electricity operates by driving and transmitting energy to an item. Crystals have the capacity to exploit energy originating from quantum sphere and deliver it to your energy field. Don't worry, unlike electricity, this mending energy is innocuous.

Balance–Our universe is very symmetrical. Look at the leaves of the shrubs or even your flesh. The energy of our planet is aligning stuff in a different model. Sometimes your energy may be misaligned and out of equilibrium and healing crystals may use the characteristics listed above, which are fundamentally attractive and repulsive, to balance out regions of vigorous disharmony.

Effective Healing Stones

1. Amethyst

Amethyst is famous for being used to heal hangovers and drunkenness. This specific crystal was proven to be useful for supporting individuals to relate to their spirituality and to enhance their psychic abilities.

The Amethyst Crystal can be particularly good for individuals with the following zodiac symbols: Pisces, Virgo, Aquarius and Capricorn.

2. Rose Quartz

The crystal is well-known as the' love glass.' This rock is widely used to attract and preserve love and to protect friendships. The Rose Quartz can also assist cure your heart of frustration and pain.

The Rose Quartz Crystal can be particularly good for Librans or Taureans.

3. Iron Pyrite

Iron Pyrite is useful to prevent any adverse energy or physical hazard you may encounter. This can also assist in making your mind and memory even more active.

The Iron Pyrite Crystal can be particularly good for Leos.

4. Tiger Eye

This crystal is highly recommended for the maintenance and growth of riches. It is also considered to assist build knowledge and consciousness and it can also be an excellent tool to use when you feel stressed, to maintain you calm.

The Tiger Eye Crystal can establish a strong connection with those born under The Capricorn sign.

5. Hematite

This specific crystal can be mainly used to bring equilibrium into your life. It could be the perfect stone to have if you're under stress and need to feel calm and focused. This precious stone can also support you in washing away any adverse emotions caused by stress or anxiety.

It is particularly useful for individuals with the following zodiac symbols: Aries and Aquarius.

6. Raw Emerald

Yet another gem that is linked to sentimental life, raw emerald is often called an 'effective love' stone. This crystal can foster concentrate, clear negativity and encourage allegiance and sensitivity.

Raw Emerald Crystal is preeminently great for people with the following zodiac signs: Taurus, Gemini and Aries.

7. Citrine

Citrine crystal highly used thanks to the comforting, utopian vibe it can emanate and it has the advantage of not having to be cleaned or recharged. This crystal also helps to prevent any adverse energy that goes in your manner.

The Citrine Crystal can be particularly good for Geminis, Aries, Libras and Leos.

8. Celestine

The crystal of Celestine can be good for soothing and balancing. Some individuals who came in contact with this crystal stated that it helped them remember their dreams. It is also able to give your body clarity and peace of mind.

Celestine Crystal is particularly helpful for Geminis.

9. Quartz Crystal

Quartz crystal is a rock with a sheer and strong source of energy. This crystal can make you feel more conscious, boost your brain and help you feel more physically active and alert. This crystal could be an excellent rock to use if you feel weary, both mentally and physically.

Quartz Crystal is that type of crystal that can work in a different way for every sign.

10. Desert Rose

This crystal is sometimes used during meditation as it is supposedly utilized as an entrance to previous and future life. It can give mental clarity as well as knowledge and consciousness to the crystal proprietor.

The Desert Rose Crystal especially connects with Taureans.

CHAPTER 9
CLEANSING YOUR CRYSTALS

Once you get a crystal, it may be fresh to you, but it's been a lengthy trip to achieve its final destination in the palms of your hands. It was taken from a mine, handed over to different handlers, who then gave it to a vendor, to sell it to a retailer, where it was touched by many customers before it was chosen by you! That's a lot of energy you don't want to operate with. Because we all want to start freshly this new journey, it is essential that the first move you take is to clean your crystals.

Luckily, there are a lot of ways to clean them and many are not only helpful for the crystals but for your mind too. From having some rest accompanied by the moonlight, or having a pleasant sound shower, these are some pleasant techniques to clean your crystals so that both you and your crystal are in the greatest purified waters. Use them every time you might feel like you need to. Same as your energy, your crystal might sometimes be congested or unanimated. In this case, you need to make sure you perform periodic purifications to make sure your crystals work at their highest potential.

Elementary means to clean your crystals

Sunlight or Moonlight Spa

Once your crystals start looking dimmed and not as animated, give them back to nature. Place them outside and let them immerse either in the moonlight or the sunlight for a couple of hours (I would suggest at least four). This process is mandatory for the bigger precious stones that you might possess, so make sure you clean them at least once every month, even if it sounds like a lot of work.

A Crystallized Cleansing with Quartz or Selenite

You can play around and perform tricks on your own. So, go ahead and match your crystals with quartz or selenite, since both have the distinctive capacity to clean, recharge and filter the energy of other crystals without reducing their energy. Place your crystals and dropped rocks on a sheet of clear quartz or a selenite charging table for 6 + hours. We like to exercise with jewelry and crystals that we use every day by placing them on the table overnight, so that in the morning they are recharged and ready to use.

When in Doubt, Smoke It Out

Not only will Sage and Frankincense burn and Palo Santo create your house smell good, but your crystals will also feel good. Immerse your crystals in the sacred smoke until it seems to be coming back to life. This is probably the greatest choice for bigger, harder crystals to pick up. Just use your feather or your fist to wave the smoke around the crystal.

Return to Nature

We could all use an effective reset of nature now and then. To give that revitalizing pleasure to your crystal, you can either leave it on the ground or bury it for a day. If you are lucky to live close to a small river or other water source, you can as well immerse your stones for some moments, making sure you do so to purify your mind. Note: be very careful when doing so, since many of the weaker crystals that are salt-based will disappear when they get moist.

How to Program Your Crystal

Just as you need a feeling of independence to be the greatest you can be, so does your crystal. Crystals will work in your favor, but you need to offer them a task. Crystals are neutral; they do not judge circumstances as excellent or bad. They're also amplifiers and when they're not programmed, they can amplify undesired things in your life–because they need to channel their power in a particular path.

Giving your crystal a task enables you to put your mind on the work you're going to do together. It produces a kind of synergy between you and your crystal partner. Get that particular! For the crystal to assist you take your conversion to light, you must be evident when programming your crystal.

> First, clean up your crystal.
> Hold it in your fingers, near your eyes and take three profound breaths through your nose and your mouth.
> Concentrate on your belief in a higher being, the Universe and on what brings you peace. This is going to link you with your greatest vibration.
> As you enter this room of strong emotion, pray for your precious stone to be freed of all undesired vibration and any prior programming. Aloud or in your brain, say: I invite you to link the greatest vibration of love and light to my greatest self to shut up all unwanted energy and any prior programming. I order this crystal to hold on to the purpose of — to complete this phrase, insert three plans for your crystal — energy that you want it to hold on to you.
> End the programming by stating thank you three times. By stating these three occasions, you stress that what you are looking for already exists in the universe.

Convenient Ways to Cleanse and Recharge Your Healing Crystals:

1. Natural Water

Water neutralizes the adverse energy stored in the rock and carries it back to the earth.

Rinse and boost your rocks with water by putting them under natural rain for a couple of minutes. If it's a dry season, you can also position your rocks in a colander and operate your rocks under a hawk for about 10 minutes.

Important to remember: Water has physical strength, so it is important to wash difficult rocks such as amethyst, turquoise, or quartz with this technique.

2. Sunlight or Moonlight

Nothing is more powerful and pure than the natural light coming from the Sun or Moon.

The sun will supply the freshly cultivated gemstone with the yang solar energy that balances the inherent energy of the stone in that it got from the earth during its development. For rocks that are prone to discoloration under the powerful sun (such as amethyst, rose quartz or amber), you can choose to bring them out for an hour at dusk.

Important to mention: Moonlight is a more sensitive (and non-color-altering) technique that is particularly efficient with the full moon, since the Moon reaches its highest capacity once it is complete.

3. Earth

Another great method that you can use to clean your crystals is by using Earth's components. So just burry the stones for 24 hours and let the soil absorb the unwanted energies that may reside in your crystals.

4. FirePower

You can use fire or smoke to clean your rocks rapidly by boiling or smudging your rocks. Direct fire instantly fires off any adverse energy and is performed over a candle in a matter of seconds. Smudging can be performed with sage stems, palo santo, or corporate incense, such as sandalwood or cedar, which is known to eliminate negativity.

Wave your rock transversely to the source for half a minute to clean it while purifying your house.

5. Salt Water

A saltwater bath is amongst the best-known ways to wash your gemstones. Throughout history, salt has been utilized in all cultures for ceremonies and as a car for the absorption of unwanted energy.

With this method, soak your rocks in water overnight with a pinch of sea salt. Ideally, if you avail of seawater, you can revive it by letting it sit in a mesh bag in the sea. Make sure that they are rinsed in transparent water after the salt shower to remove any residue.

Important to remember: it is not always advisable to use salt water to clean the rocks, as some sensitive materials such as hematite or pyrite may be damaged by salt.

6. Other Stones

Some particular crystals and rock congregate (such as quartz or amethyst) can absorb and regenerate other rocks. Selenite is one of the most widely used purification crystals that can purify gemstones from their negativity.

To clean your stones, place them on a selenite surface for at least 6 hours (but the longer, the better). Selenite and transparent quartz clusters effectively amplify the vibration in other crystals. They can absorb, neutralize and then recharge your rocks with greater temperatures.

7. Meditation

Yes, you can meditate on your manner to cleared rocks! At the same moment, there are methods to wash and meditate on your gemstones.

During meditation, you can balance your energies by drawing a healthy breath on your gems. It's essential to state your desire so that after you wash it, you can refuel your gemstone. If you exercise this type of crystal purification regularly, it will come naturally. And once you reach your peace of mind you will be able to perform this type of meditation easily.

Please notice: do not do this in vain. Make sure you exercise this with relaxed, real meditation. The double whammy is to do a meditation-cleaning on a full moon!

Whether you're in the market for a fresh stone to add to your collection or want to learn how to keep your current stones, it's essential to purify them frequently.

The color, texture and sensation of rock perform a major part in expressing a season, a Chakra and–also–your character.

CHAPTER 10
HOW TO UTILIZE CRYSTAL BALLS: STEP BY STEP GUIDE

The crystal ball appears in numerous films, television displays, comics and even pictures about psychic mediums and fortune-telling. You might even have seen one on a monument inside a half of a fortune teller machine in a theme park. But the crystal ball is far more than a prop.

Mastering the crystal ball use can be an interesting method for many, but also one full of embarrassment. You may never have taken a course at college on how to use one, but there are still tips and tricks that are essential to understand!

Whether you're extending your work as a psychic medium or wanting to delve deeper into teaching about the craft as a whole, reading a little about the crystal ball is an appropriate way to get started. Here, we're going to explain the structure and work of the mystical crystal ball, as well as how you can learn to look at the crystal ball and use it to perceive signals about the future.

The Functions of a Crystal Ball

The first thing you understand about your crystal ball is precisely what it's capable of. It is not only about looking into the future. It can also function as a conduit to increase a particular sort of vibration in the region. These ideas that you stimulate can be anything from reconciliation to romance. Its spherical form makes it possible to cast this energy in many ways that is component of what makes it so strong.

The function of the crystal ball can be enhanced based on the fabric. Some products are better for screaming, which implies looking at the ball for psychic reasons. Some are better at boosting distinct kinds of energy.

> ➢ Rose Quartz is good for romance

> ➢ Rhodonite is great for reconciliation

> ➢ Moonstone / Red Silicone increases Passion

> ➢ Hermitage takes your relationships to another level

> ➢ Sunstone Exudes Sexuality

By using a crystal ball, you can carry meditation sessions, as well as other religious conferences or sessions. The opportunities of what you can do with it are infinite, but the material is a significant consideration to consider.

This implies that it's essential to think about what you'd like the role of your crystal ball to be before you buy it. Reflect, study and then decide.

How to care for your Crystal Ball

Among the most complex variables to consider when buying a crystal ball is how to preserve it. Since it has a spherical shape, it diffuses energy in many directions, so it may be mind-boggling to think about how you could potentially store and regulate this power.

There are many methods to pay your crystal ball before a meeting, some of which include placing it, placing it in the moonlight, or cleaning it in holy water or incense smoke. These techniques of loading the ball enable the vibration of the earth, the cosmos, the incense and the holy water to be absorbed.

It is vital to charge your crystal ball before reading. It cleans up previous meetings and guarantees that the energy is free and not exhausted. The way you chose to store the balls is incredibly important for this purpose too. It is vital to store it out of sight in a dark cabinet where it can rest.

Preparing for a Crystal Ball Reading

Prep job is not just about the crystal ball. You need to clean up your crystal ball as well as the atmosphere and your state of mind. Purify your mind in the manner you're going to have your crystal ball. The finest technique for your mind is meditation or stimulating operations that assist you in reaching the peak of the head.

If you go into reading with wild feelings or other ideas that distract you, it will most probably contribute to bad reading. Crystal ball screaming is already hard; you don't want to make it harder for yourself by being inattentive and negligent.

The workplace is also essential to be part of the equation. It is essential to keep the lighting dim so that not too much light is reflected from the crystal ball and to keep the noise out or to a minimum. Make sure the devices are ignored or off and distractions are left out of the house.

Once you, space and the ball have been cleaned and correctly taken care of, you're prepared to start screaming at your crystal ball.

How To Use A Crystal Ball

No matter how it appears in the films, crystal ball screaming is more than just waving your arms above the crystal ball and announcing someone's future. The method requires years of training to be prepared to conduct an insightful study.

One of the essential elements to concentrate on during reading is the power of the sphere. This little ball is designed to be rounded, in order to propagate energy all around it. This implies that channeling and reacting to that energy is crucial if you accept what the crystal ball has to give you as a medium.

Step 1: Charging Ball

Holding the pen before reading is a lovely method to link your energy to the crystal ball. As you cleaned it just before the meeting, it now carries the divine or natural energy that you have loaded, as well as your energy.

Step 2: Set Ball to Flat Surface Facing You

Start by putting it down to whatever you've set to the table for you. It could be a stand or a cloth, or just a set. A stack may operate best so that the object does not spin or drop.

Step 3: Looking at The Ball

Remember sooner when you meditated and removed your mind? Well, it's not just component of the training method. Meditation is the fundamental way that offers the opportunity to tap into the energy that the crystal ball is carrying off.

Clearing your mind of distractions allows you to focus on any texts that the crystal ball may be displaying you. Start by looking at the crystal ball and trying to concentrate on the box, ridding your mind of other distractions.

Step 4: Mist Begins To Form

Once your concentration and concentrate have reached an important level, you will see a fog starting to develop. An error many beginners create is that when they lastly start to see the fog, they panic or get enthusiastic and lose concentration.

Step 5: Images Begin To Reveal Themselves

Instead of enabling the sight of the fog to lead you to panic, be ready for it instead and proceed to concentrate. After a time of uninterrupted concentration, pictures and texts will start to disclose themselves to you in the fog.

It's difficult to define what these posts might be because they're distinct for everyone. It is most probable to arrive in the shape of colors, forms, phrases and signs. You might also feel this vibration on your body.

Interpreting Symbols and Messages

It is not necessarily easy to interpret these posts. You're not always going to have an entire situation before you perform. Most of the time, you're going to have to determine what several seemingly nonsensical images teach you about the future.

Practice making sense of these pictures by focusing on understanding the vibrations you get. How do you feel about these signs? What are they going to make you believe of? Take the filter off your perceptive, analytical abilities and bring all the data and try to see how it fits together.

Think about these issues as you try to understand the symbols:

> ➢ How do these symbols create me feel?
>
> ➢ Are those signs linked to each other?
>
> ➢ What kind of electricity do the signs give off?

As you deal with these issues and the responses to them, try to link together the possible narratives or situations that these signs might be related to. If you stay concentrated, more and more clarity will come to you in a moment. In the original efforts to scrip though, you may have a very random-seeking range of emails that can be difficult to create sense of.

Be Patient With Yourself

The road you need to take in order to be trained to operate correctly as a medium that uses a crystal ball is a lengthy one, but it is also filled with thrill and exciting discoveries. It can be simple to get bored with how hard it is to maintain concentrate and obtain psychic inputs from the crystal ball, so it is essential to acknowledge that this capacity develops with the moment.

Don't give up right away just because you're having difficulty seeing anything in the bag. Just maintain concentrating and looking, be careful in your prep job and over the moment, you'll ultimately find that your skills have expanded and you'll be able to see more as you look at the crystal ball.

We're all growing at distinct prices. We're all learning at distinct speeds. Being tough on yourself can only slow you down on your path to becoming a psychic medium. Be patient and accept yourself to move forward and proceed to learn utilizing a glass ball.

CHAPTER 11
SIMPLE INTRODUCTION TO CHAKRA

hakras may appear to be an airy-fairy and all' fresh ages.' When you start to know about them, you can see how much they call to inform us about ourselves.

In the Yoga tradition, the human body has seven energy centers called Chakras. When these power centers are safe and accessible, so are we— physically, emotionally, mentally and in our interactions with ourselves and others. But when they're prevented by accident, disease, or disconnection from others, we're prevented from being our greatest self and can feel annoyed, trapped and lacking in vitality.

Throughout our adolescence and through our lives experiences, we often generate constrictions in our Chakras. For example, if we were constantly criticized for our chants, we could shut down our fifth Chakra (neck center) by restricting our artistic speech or capacity to talk up for ourselves.

Traumas, concerns and' adverse' feelings can contribute to long-term imbalances in your energy system, resulting in difficulties such as insecurity, rage, stress, or disease.

We often attempt to comprehend ourselves better through Western psychology, which is fantastic, but sometimes an essential element–our energy scheme–is lacking. It is also essential to tackle our fundamental energy system, which impacts how we live, breathe and communicate ourselves.

This is where healing energy goes in. It promotes a vigorous scheme to clean up constrictions in your environment that may have an impact on your life force in tens of respects.

How to understand if my seven Chakras are in equilibrium?

Our organs are in the steady flux of equilibrium and imbalance. Balance is not static; it's always shifting. Awareness is the starting point, as once you introduce consciousness to your body/mind, you can begin learning its hints and hints. You start to hear to your body at all stages as your guide.

When we think nice, comfortable and happy in the globe, then our energy is moving, we feel like we're in the stream. However, if we feel depressed, nervous, strained and so on, our energy will be exhausted and our amount of vitality may also be impacted. Over moment, this will influence the well-being of a person and this is where Reiki or Shamanic Healing would be very useful.

We live in a globe where the pace seems to be growing quicker, almost to the stage where we're going for twenty-four-seven, or where we think we should be. As we move forward in our lives, the majority of us tend to lose balance and harmony.

Instead of choosing to enjoy every day and to be grateful for everything that life has gifted us with, we are concerned about the past and the future and let the present pass by. All this concern and stress in our regular life impacts our energy centers and they become closed, i.e. the energy does not pass freely through the Chakras.

A' block' is a location where energy is caught or constrained. In coping with a block, you need to move the energy that Reiki does. When energy moves through the whole body, it generates harmony and generates imbalances. Reiki helps put the Chakras into alignment and equilibrium.

No Chakra operates separately of the other Chakras and they are all component of the entire energy system. Each Chakra only operates fully when the other Chakras are fully involved. They're all component of the whole thing.

Every one of the seven Chakras plays a role in maintaining some part of our lives physically, emotionally, mentally, or spiritually.

Many things affect our Chakras, from our physical setting to our feelings to our emotional conversation. It is vital for excellent health to be conscious of how balanced or unbalanced our Chakras are.

What is Energy?

Energy is our life force if we are to accomplish all that we want, then we need to maximize our energy levels. The greater your energy levels, the easier you feel and the more likely you are to accomplish your outcomes, as you bring all your' energy' into it. In Japan, energy is called' Ki,' meaning universal power of existence.

Energy flows continuously through our body and in many healing aspects, it is described as travelling through all seven vibration centers, or through our Chakras, even though we don't physically see it.

Energy is something we can all sense, but most of us think it unconsciously.

Close your eyes and try reminiscing a moment when you felt happy observing a lovely sunrise. Observe how you start feeling while imagining this. You might discover that you begin laughing, that you feel warmth in your core, or that you feel peace in your stomach.

On the other side, remember the task you had with a college or spouse. Notice how you feel while remembering this scene. You may discover that you feel close around your neck that your heart beats high, that your palm sweats and that you feel nervous.

Have you noticed the distinction in what you've been feeling? While you're talking about a scenario you've liked feeling relaxed, stuff flow and time move rapidly. However, once you start remembering the dispute, you probably felt tense, anxious, suffocated, out of balance. You react in this way as your body is responding to the energy, thoughts and emotions.

Energy Loves Flowing

Simply talking, if you even believe about something that's bothering you, you're likely sick of attempting to figure it out, many of you feel a knot in your stomach, rage growing from the inside or trapped as you can see the wood from the forests.

From this place, it can be more difficult to make decisions that feel matched–this is where healing goes in.

Energy likes to pass and wants to move, but it can get stuck. This is when you need healing, in order to facilitate the energy flow through the body so that you don't get 'lost' in the feelings.

The Main Aspects of the 7 Chakras

Root Chakra

The' root Chakra' is situated at the core of the vertebral column, forming our basis. It reflects the composition of the Earth and is linked to our survival instincts (food, refuge and security). It stimulates us to handle ourselves gently and sustain ourselves, encouraging our survival instincts.

It speaks to our capacity of being grounded and in touch with our physical bodies and the physical universe. Ideally, the Root Chakra gives us safety and existence here and now. It shows us what we need to survive. It is the basis of our faith in the material world.

The sense of fear is one of the main forces affecting the root Chakra. The archetypes of the root Chakra are Mother and Victim.

Sacral Chakra

The' sacral Chakra' is known to be found in the abdomen, upper lip and sexual organs. It concerns the component of water and our feelings and sexuality. Its primary role is to give us a feeling of self–our internal self / inner baby. It's the origin of creativity and inspiration. This Chakra regulates our appetite for feeling, whether it's through noise, smell, taste, touch or vision.

It confers us deep feelings, sexual satisfaction and the capacity to embrace change. It gives us up to what we seek and it enables us to revel in the nature and delight of existence, it manifests for us what we seek and what gives us enjoyment.

One of the most influential forces to affect the sacred Chakra is guilt. The archetypes of the sacred Chakra are the Emperor / Empress and the Martyr.

Solar Plexus

The 'solar plexus ' Chakra is regarded as the 'energy Chakra' situated on the solar plexus. Its primary role is to deliver energy through warmth, vitality and excitement. It governs our awareness of decision-making, artistic expression, personal power, will and self-determination and it also affects or metabolism. When we are in equilibrium, we have good self-esteem, trust, self-esteem and are willing to create choices by ourselves.

Honesty represents one of the attributes that influence the solar plexus. The archetypes of the solar plexus are the peaceful warrior and the servant.

Heart Chakra

The 'heart Chakra' is situated in the middle of your neck. It's about love and compassion. The Chakra links the reduced ego / physical self with the greater soul / spiritual self. It helps to take joy to us by handing out love and it attracts what we enjoy into our life. In equilibrium, our fourth Chakra enables us to enjoy profoundly, to feel compassion and to feel a profound feeling of peace and focus. We're allowing ourselves to love unconditionally.

Grief is among the main elements that influence the heart Chakra. The lover and the actor are the prototypes that characterize the heart Chakra.

Throat Chakra

This Chakra can be found in the neck area, as it is linked to interaction, self-expression and creativity. As we rediscover our personal & genuine self, it enables us to convey ourselves, to communicate obviously what we need, think, willingness and thinks. It enables free communication to help us feel focused and pleased. It also enables us as we meditate to communicate with our greater guidelines. The Chakra is directly connected to your inner self, deeply linked to your soul and enables you to hear as your soul talks.

Dishonesty is one of the main tendencies that influence the throat Chakra. The Communicator and the Silent Child are the archetypes of the throat Chakra.

Third Eye

This Chakra is regarded as the brow Chakra or the third eye. It is situated slightly above and between the brows. Its primary role is being the source of inner vision. The third eye is the location of intuition and understanding of the soul. As such, it opens up our faculties of psychic and spiritual consciousness along with our knowledge of archetypal dimensions. When we're in equilibrium, it enables us to have an understanding. It teaches us the authority of the mind to assist us ' dream large' and to build our required truth.

An illusion represents one of the main elements affecting the third eye Chakra. Its archetypes are the Intuitive and the Intellectual.

Crown Chakra

The 'crown Chakra' refers to consciousness as sheer awareness. It's situated at the base of the head. It is our link to the collective consciousness and the wider globe beyond. It is thought that this is where the soul joins the physical body at birth and leaves once we are dead. When in equilibrium and working at its full potential, this Chakra brings us comprehension, insight, awareness, spiritual connection and harmony. It opens our eyes to the fact that we are spiritual entities, links us to the holy dimension and helps us to experience being "one with all that is".

Attachment represents one of the main feelings directly affecting the crown Chakra. The perfect specimens of the crown Chakra are the Guru and the Egot

CHAPTER 12
THE BASIS OF REIKI

Reiki is an alternative therapy frequently referred to as energy cure. It arose in Japan in the late 1800s and is said to involve the transition of universal energy from the practitioner's palms to the individual.

Energy mending has been practiced in various forms for centuries. Advocates claim it works with the power ranges around the body.

There have always been controversaries surrounding Reiki because it is difficult to demonstrate its efficacy by scientific means. However, many individuals who tried Reiki claim it really works, so lately its fame is on an ascending scale. Google's query for the word presently yields no less than 68,900,000 outcomes.

A 2007 survey shows that 1,2 million adults in America (U.S.) had tried Reiki or similar therapy once or more in the past year. Also, there are numerous therapy centers known to offer Reiki, as well as many hospitals (around 60).

Some quick details about Reiki

We are going to list some of the main aspects regarding Reiki more details to be debated in the dedicated chapter.

Reiki is a mending practice.

> ➢ Despite skepticism in some circles, popularity is growing.

> ➢ It is based on a technique known as "laying on of hands", which involves an energy transfer from the healer to the patient.

> ➢ Reiki proponents affirm that they are able to handle many circumstances and mental states.

> ➢ Small trials indicate that Reiki can decrease suffering mildly, but no trials have shown that it is efficient in handling any disease.

> ➢ Reiki is offered by some clinics in America and Europe, but insurance scarcely includes it.

What is Reiki?

The term "Reiki" stands for "mysterious atmosphere, miraculous sign." It comes from the Japanese words "rei" (universal) and "ki" (life energy). Reiki is a kind of healing energy.

This energy mending targets the power fields in our bodies.

According to practitioners, energy may clog the areas of our body where we had injuries or, possibly, emotional pain. These energy blockages can affect us in time, by causing illnesses.

The objective of a Reiki session is to release the blocked energy the same manner acupuncture does. Improving the energy flux around the body, claim professionals, can help to relax, decrease pain, speed up recovery and decrease other signs of disease.

Reiki existed for thousands of years now. Its present type was first created in 1922 by a Japanese Buddhist named Mikao Usui, who supposedly instructed 2,000 Americans the Reiki technique during his lifetime. The practice started spreading to the United States through Hawaii in the 1940s and lately, it reached Europe around the 1980s.

It is commonly mentioned as hand healing or palm healing.

What happens in a Reiki session?

Reiki is best kept in a serene environment, but it can be performed out anywhere. The patient usually seats in a cozy seat, or lays on a table, fully dressed. Music may or may not be played, depending on the preference of the patient.

The person puts his palms gently on or over particular regions of the head, arms and torso, using separate forms of the hand, for 2 to 5 minutes. Hands can be put over 20 distinct parts of the body.

If there is a specific injury, such as a burn, the hands may be held just above the wound.

As the healer lightly positions his hands on or over the body, the energy transfer takes place. During this time, the hands of the practitioner may be warm and tingling. Each hand position is kept until the physician feels that the energy has ceased flowing.

When the physician thinks that the heat or energy in their hands has faded, they will remove their palms and position them over a distinct region of the body.

Some Reiki methods the methods concerned have names such as:

- ➤ centering
- ➤ clearing
- ➤ beaming
- ➤ extracting damaging energies
- ➤ infusing
- ➤ smoothing and raking the aura

Some Reiki professionals use crystals and Chakra purification wands because they discover that they can heal or safeguard the house from adverse electricity.

Health benefits

According to professionals, therapeutic impacts are transmitted by channeling the natural energy recognized as qi, called "chi." In India, it is called "prana." It's the same power engaged in tai chi practice. It's the energy of life force that some think surrounds us all.

The energy is said to permeate the body. Experts from Reiki point out that while this energy is not measurable by contemporary science methods, it can be felt by many who plug into it.

Reiki is said to help relax, help in the natural healing procedures of the body and establish physical, psychical and spiritual wellness.

It was also proven to induce profound relaxation, to assist individuals to deal with problems, alleviate emotional stress and enhance general well-being.

Individuals who have experienced the healing power of Reiki, often describe it as profoundly unwinding. Reiki was proven to help treating numerous conditions as:

- Cancer
- Heart diseases
- Anxiety
- Depression
- Chronic pain
- Infertility
- Neurodegenerative disorders
- Autism
- Crohn's disease
- Fatigue syndrome.

CHAPTER 13
PENDULUM DOWSING AN INITIATION TO USING A PENDULUM

Among the most frequently utilized divination and dowsing instruments is the pendulum. Mastering a pendulum is a skill that anyone can achieve, being a really enjoyable practice. Here's an introduction to using a pendulum, how it operates and what you need in order to start.

First, what is a pendulum?

The pendulum is an asymmetrical, weighted item suspended from a single chain or wire. It's never produced of a magnetic material, but it's often made of crystal. It is also feasible to use items such as a stone, a metallic ball, a bead or a button. The pendulum is a very easy instrument that allows the customer to adjust to their intuitive forces. The pendulum functions as a receiver and transmitter of data and travels in a wide range of directions to answer questions.

What Is Pendulum Dowsing Used For?

This technique can be used in some different approaches. In its simplest shape, you can use it to reply questions or help in decision-making. Pendulums can also be utilized in:

> ➤ Healing and allergy identification reasons.

> ➤ Clean up and dispel the negativity in the space.

> ➤ Help you discover missed items or animals.

> ➤ To discover water or law rows (the dowsing wheels that operate comparably to the pendulum are often used for this purpose).

What Is The Technique Behind Pendulum Dowsing?

The pendulum operates by pushing into your instinct and your sixth sense. It functions as a type of receiver and transmitter, through your greater supervision, guardian angels and religious educators. As the pendulum shifts, you get responses to issues—it's best to use to reply' yes' or' no' questions. Some individuals define how the pendulum operates as putting together the rational and spontaneous side of you (the left and the correct side of your brain). When both of these elements are put together, you can create choices using all the sources, rather than just one of them.

Where are the answers coming from?

Many individuals ask were the responses originate from and discuss whether they work, or just the pendulum that responds to the motion of the user's side. You can certainly make the instrument move by simply using your hand force, this isn't always the situation and after exercise, you'll see why. As with any divination, the use of the pendulum requires a certain amount of faith, belief and an unequivocally oppenness, as the responses originate from your intuition and greater religious guides.

What Sort of Pendulum Do I Need?

There are many types of pendulums available for dowsing, but you certainly don't have to purchase a smart, costly pendulum to get a nice result. In reality, the sort of pendulum you choose relies, in portion, on what you feel correct about. The majority of individuals opt for crystal pendulums. Clear quartz, for instance, is a common option, as this gemstone is associated to clarity and a greater intent. Amethyst, which has a strong connection to the spiritual, is often common, as is a pendulum with the calming characteristics of a rose quartz crystal.

After all, as long as it is rounded or pointed at one end, doesn't matter if you chose based on your instinct or rationality. Furthermore, if you prefer to, you can also combine different crystals and have more than one pendulum. When you get started, you could train on basic concepts using a do-it-yourself pendulum or a handmade pendulum if you want. You could use, for example, a spherical bead made of glass, a metallic ball, or even a key attached at the end of a string. Once you realize that you've mastered this craft to some extent, you can switch to a more meticulously designed pendulum.

Before using a pendulum

Before every use of a pendulum, it is advisable to clean it and fill it with your vibration. The most uncomplicated way to clean your dowsing pendulum is to put it on the windowsill in direct sunlight for a day to catch the sun's rays. To supply it with your energy, keep the pendulum in your fingers and close your fingers around it. Then spend a short time (5 to 15 minutes will be all right) sitting softly, your eyes shut, concentrating your energy on your pendulum. If you would like to, you can recite an invocation or ask your spiritual guides or guardian angels for their assistance and advice when using the pendulum. Once your pendulum is cleaned and loaded, it's a good idea to maintain it secure. A lot of individuals like to wrap their pendulums in silk or pop them in a tiny velvet sack to keep them safe.

How to Get Started With Using a Pendulum

Anyone can use a pendulum, but the primary criterion is that you must begin with an open mind and placed any doubts on one hand. The string, loop, or should be held between the thumb and the forefinger in which the hand feels most relaxed. Some pendulums have a tiny metal loop or ring at the base of the string that can render it simple to maintain. Ideally, the pendulum chain shouldn't be too long, particularly when you first start, so if it seems too long or you have a surplus string or chord, you can tie it around your index finger gently.

Once you feel prepared to get started, hold your pendulum between your thumb and your index finger and move the other hand over the entire length of the chain or rope, bringing your hand to rest with the lower tip of the pendulum in your upturned palm. Now the pendulum needs to be still and you can push your hand back from the top of the pendulum. As you push it back, the pendulum is likely to begin swinging. This is completely ordinary.

Try and be as relaxed as possible (the higher the level of relaxation, the better the energy flux) and observe the pendulum movement while you stay seated peacefully. While doing this, start examining the rhythm, the way the pendulum stops so that you can learn to read the "yes" and "no" signals. At this point, you can try asking your pendulum out loud or in your mind to give you a "yes" response. Take a little while to observe the reaction–it may be very superficial at first, but don't worry, because this is normal, as it takes time both for you and the pendulum to learn how to interact with each other.

Take a small break and allow your energy to be balanced before asking you pendulum for a "no". Don't worry if you can't tell much difference from the yes and no responses yet –this is perfectly normal at first and you should get to be able to tell the difference with time and practice. For example, many pendulums will answer "yes" by following a wide, rounded movement while in case of a "no" you will be able to distinguish more of a back and forth flow.

You will need to repeat this exercise numerous times until getting used to the way the pendulum responds. The "yes" e "no" responses vary based on the vibes you transfer to the pendulum and, moreover, they will obviously vary based on the person who's asking. So, in case someone else used your pendulum, you will need to recharge it with your energy, to reestablish the familiar bond.

What Type of Questions Can I Ask the Pendulum?

The pendulum responds better to questions where there are "yes" or "no" answers. Begin with simple questions, as "Is today Tuesday?", "Is my best friend's name Phil?" or "Am I based in Italy?". This will facilitate the understanding of the pendulum's reactions and will help you to better connect with it, in order to comprehend each other. As you become more dexterous with your pendulum, you can start counting on it regarding life decision, such as buying a new piece of furniture for your house, choosing a healthier diet or deciding if you can trust a certain individual in your life. But the abilities of the pendulum could be used in fun ways too. Do not feel limited to serious issues. Go ahead and use your pendulum to guide you to a castle or a water source on a map. Move it over the map and see the reactions. In time, with more experience, you will also be able to use this method to find people or animals.

What If My Pendulum Doesn't Work?

There are some cases where your pendulum might not operate, or you might get the incorrect answers to your issues.

> You may have misinterpreted the' yes' and' no' motions of your pendulum for several purposes.
> If you are attempted, angry, mental or feeling out of color, it may not operate correctly.
> If you are not comfortable enough or feel negative.
> You may be too near to high-frequency electrical equipment or machinery that could influence your pendulum.
> You have not phrased your requests correctly–they need to be easy and particular.
> You don't concentrate enough–sometimes you have to wait a while for the response to pass through.
> You might want to attempt using a distinct pendulum, as it may not be consistent with your energy.

CHAPTER 14
QUARTZ CRYSTALS

Quartz crystals are made of silica (scientifically known as silicone dioxide) and can be found in a wide range of shapes and shades. Many are transparent or translucent.

They come in a variety of appealing colors and the majority of them have strong healing properties. Their characteristics are quite varied and many have powerful vibrations.

Quartz has many excellent qualities, among which the ability to be programmed, detail that makes it a very powerful stone, able to help you manifest the life you desire.

Quartz is used by sector because of its piezoelectric characteristics and its amplification characteristics.

It is this particular quality that makes these stones very powerful for metaphysical reasons and produces strong healing properties within the stones.

Where are they coming from?

Quartz Meaning

The name quartz originates from the ancient Anglo-Saxon term "Quartz" which means "rock crystal".

They are the most prolific form of crystals discovered on Earth and because of the vastity of types and shapes, they exist all over the globe.

Many of the quartz parts you see have a classic prismatic form. The record holder crystal shown further down this section is an instance of the classic quartz form of all kinds.

As we stated, these crystals develop in many forms, from huge bits of rock to small crystals on the matrix. However, based on the specific type and where it comes from, they can grow in different ways.

Each of the distinct kinds of quartz may have distinct inclusions within the fundamental quartz framework, which adds to the distinctive color and vibration of each quartz form.

This implies that inclusions generate unique metaphysical characteristics, which is why quartz has so many differences insignificance.

Many distinct quartz settings and structures also produce characteristics that render them strong for use both in your regular lives and for healing, so it's worth learning before you choose your crystal.

There are also enormous differences in their increasing practices, which implies that you may discover them rising naturally in the location where you reside.

Wearing Quartz Crystals

Any kind of quartz is lovely to carry as it guides the energy flow where is more needed. Wearing a lovely piece of jewelry that is also such a powerful healing instrument is very helpful.

This item involves three distinct quartz crystals, the light purple Citrine, the Purple Amethyst and the beautiful Ametrine stone, all in one pendant.

Ametrine is quite striking, as it is a blend formed with two different shades and many quartz crystals have very vivid colors.

Beautiful quartz pendants can be bought in many distinct colors, such as the vivid Harlequin Quartz, which is very appealing.

The mixture of powerful healing characteristics and lovely stones places quartz jewelry among the most popular.

Your aura will absorb energy from any natural crystal that you might wear (rings, pendants etc.). This implies that you are continually able to use the vibration they emit.

Amethyst clusters can be used to help you clean your jewelry. Place your necklace or pendant on a stack of beautiful Amethyst Crystals overnight to clean it up of negativity.

How to use that... Why would you be using it?

Between the most beautiful varieties of quartz we can distinguish Yellow Citrine, Pink Rose Quartz, Purple Amethyst and the astonishing Golden Healer Quartz.

If you want to add one to your collection, you will be able to choose from a huge range of quartz crystals, with different attributes.

Using a pendulum is now a well-known therapeutic method, as it provides the user with immediate feedback on the issue. Pendulums are great instruments to ensure you get responses from the spirit.

Although the pendulums are produced by a multitude of distinct rocks, the quartz pendulums are quite strong owing to their amplification characteristics and are easy to purchase.

Beautiful crystal bowls are produced of distinct kinds of quartz crystals, although they are widely used in white quartz. They are especially used as a way to store precious stones.

Clear or white crystals are very common and come in many distinct settings, like this exciting record keeper shown below. Clear quartz can be made of crystal wands.

These are produced of transparent quartz, which can be precisely sliced into strong Vogel wands. Vogels are powerful metaphysical healing instruments that provide a vaster volume of healing energy.

Quartz May Be Utilized to Heal Yourself & Others

Just getting a crystals cluster in the space is powerful owing to its powerful amplification characteristics. Their vibration will echo outward, both in the room where they are located and in the nearby rooms.

Quartz crystals are often utilized for regeneration in body layouts, either by putting rocks on the body or around the body.

As their energy resonates so strongly, they don't have to touch your body to produce a healthy healing result.

Healers will usually position parts of quartz in the Chakras to help to heal. They may be put on the table close the individual being cured or even under the table and they may not have to be in direct contact with the body to operate.

High Vibration Quartz Crystals

Many types of quartz will help you connect to angels. These include rocks such as Elestial Quartz, Angel Phantom Quartz, widely known as Amphibole Quartz, Ajoite Quartz, Angel Aura Quartz, Lemurian Seed Crystals and Herkimer Diamonds.

Some quartz crystals have a large amount of crystal energy and are shown on a website devoted to high-vibration crystals.

Because they embody the quartz characteristic to amplify their energy and are of elevated vibration, this allows the use of these powerful rocks to help your private voyage.

Herkimer Diamonds possess a beautiful energy that is strong to mix with scarce or low-vibration diamonds.

This mixture can be useful if you use lower rocks in your regular crystal meditation.

You can also choose from other high-vibration quartz crystals such as Nirvana Quartz, Black Star Quartz, Dream Quartz, Rainbow Quartz, Satyaloka Quartz, Fire Quartz aka Ignite or Golden Healer.

Quartz Clusters are very beneficial.

Many kinds of quartz have great healing characteristics, which is why quartz crystal massage is so common.

A quartz cluster has the capacity of amplifying the good energy in the area where it is kept.

The purple flame healing energy is reflected in the Purple Amethyst Crystals and these lovely crystals are amazing healing tools.

This can be an outstanding healing instrument that does not require any effort on your behalf. Beautiful lavender and purple amethyst clusters have fantastic energy and are strong in every space.

Every species of quartz has the capability of elevating the perspective of the individuals using it, with the condition of being programmed to do so.

Quarts crystals energy is also widely used by healers, to better perform their healing techniques and ensure improved results..

.

CHAPTER 15
TOURMALINE CRYSTAL

Tourmaline is a highly protective stone present in many forms, all renowned for their efficiency on grounding their holder and protecting them from damaging psychic energies.

Although Tourmaline can be discovered worldwide, it is nevertheless slightly less common and much sought-after.

The rarity of Tourmaline Crystals is a consequence of the circumstances they crystallize in: they tend to take shape in compact stones, as quartz or granite.

Having an elongated and thin shape makes Tourmaline Crystals very fragile and therefore, difficult to extract whole.

It is therefore prevalent to discover Tourmaline Crystal in tiny bits and pieces that are comparatively cheap.

Complete, continuous Tourmaline Crystal wands are much more hard to locate and are therefore much more costly.

The popularity of Tourmaline started in 1876 when the mineralogist George Kunz donated a sample of Green Tourmaline to Tiffany and the New York Company.

Today, Tourmaline is recognized by mystical professionals who use it for its vigorous and protective characteristics.

Tourmaline Crystal Meaning

Known as the Grounding Stone, the Tourmaline Crystal is a highly secure stone that is commonly used by Shamanic professionals for ritual safety.

The earthing energy of Tourmaline turns it into a powerful equilibrium source, a bridge between mind and flesh.

Tourmaline Crystals are also widely used for scrying, a magical type of remote viewing performed by Aztec shamans.

The power of Tourmaline Crystal makes it the ideal meditation stone, being able to help you connect with Mother Earth and also root into your being.

The vigorous characteristics of Tourmaline assist us to progress beyond our constraints, transcending private practices and the tendency to understand our private aspirations.

The term Tourmaline is obtained from the old Sinhalese word' turmoil,' meaning precious stone of many colors.

The term' turmoil' also implies' something tiny from Earth.' Tourmaline Crystal

Properties

Among the most convincing and useful characteristics is its capacity to perform electrical charges and thus become energized. So, when it is either heated or rubbed, tourmaline charges with electricity.

Alchemists often concluded that tourmaline is linked to the philosophical stone because of its pyroelectric properties.

When loaded, the Tourmaline Crystal is fundamentally polarized, one end is positive and the other negative, providing it the capacity to attract or repel dust particles and ash.

In the 1700s, Dutch traders used Tourmaline Crystals to capture and repel ash and dust.

Tourmaline belongs to a class of compounds recognized as borosilicates of aluminum.

The level of purity is determined by the color that the particular tourmaline crystal has. It can be mixed with other metals in a lower or higher proportion.

Tourmaline Crystals are prismatic, striated crystals with a vertical framework that can develop like dense pillars or slender, striated leaves in the adjacent rock.

Natural Tourmaline Crystal wands are great for cleaning the aura of a person and for maintaining the meridian system of the body.

Varieties of Tourmaline and Their Properties

Tourmaline (Black)

95% of all Tourmaline discovered in the natural universe is Black Tourmaline, also recognized as Shorl.

Repelling negativity, Black Tourmaline raises dark moods its bases being in the Earth's power.

Blue Tourmaline

Blue Tourmaline awakens the third eye and neck Chakras, helping us to retrieve greater understanding and internal enlightenment.

Green Tourmaline

Linked to the Heart Chakra, this type of tourmaline has the ability to connect our brain to the third eye, creating a bond between our rational being and the intuitive, spiritual one.

Green Tourmaline opens our lives to others, showing us compassion and bringing wealth and abundance.

Pink Tourmaline

Pink Tourmaline opens up the Heart Chakra, encouraging emotions of happiness and love.

Pink Tourmaline is the perfect crystal for individuals who are suffering from violence.

Red Tourmaline

This particular tourmaline has direct effects on the root Chakra, improving the energy and vitality of the body.

Tourmaline Quartz

Needles and pillars of Black Tourmaline can be discovered enclosed in crystals of plain, transparent Quartz, which appear to be caught inside.

Tourmaline Quartz helps to deflect adverse electrons and activate energy blockages in the body, allowing the fluids to flow freely within us.

Watermelon Tourmaline

A very particular stone, Watermelon Tourmaline can be bought in "pieces" of Pink Tourmaline encircled by "rind" or Green Tourmaline.

Watermelon Tourmaline encourages unconditional love, binds the heart Chakra to the vibration of the higher self and brings levity and empathy.

Tourmaline Mending Features

Tourmaline wands are believed to have supernatural abilities to carry healing and light into the life of all who are attracted to them.

Tourmaline gives equilibrium, healing and alignment to our energy system.

Physical Healing

Tourmaline's extremely protective energy protects the body from debilitating illnesses by enhancing and enhancing the immune system.

Tourmaline is also useful in boosting the nervous system, re-aligning the spinal column and boosting the reflex points in the lower back, legs, wrists and legs.

Tourmaline is an outstanding pain-reducing agent that relieves circumstances such as broken joints, numbness, joint pain and arthritis.

Black Tourmaline is efficient in treating a range of digestive issues, relieving constipation, IBS and colon disorders.

Tourmaline also provides restorative and purifying characteristics, releasing heavy metals and environmental toxins from the body.

Tourmaline is the ideal instrument to restore cognitive functioning by balancing the functioning of the brain hemispheres.

This puts all our cognitive processes in connection with the etheric energy of our aura.

A healthy brain and supercharged nervous system increase hand and eye cooperation, assisting individuals to conquer anxiety, paranoia and even dyslexia.

Emotional Healing

Tourmaline cleanses our adverse ideas and disturbing emotions, such as anxiety, rage and feelings of indignity.

The grounding impact of Tourmaline Crystal helps to balance our moods, assisting us to solve suicidal thoughts, substance abuse issues and self-destructive behaviors.

Tourmaline can also relieve obsessive ideas, free individuals from OCD symptoms, obsessive anxiety and compulsive behavior.

Once released from concern and negative ideas, we discover ourselves free from the adverse impacts of stress, capable of dealing with circumstances without spiraling out of control.

Tourmaline also banishes doubts and bad ideas, encouraging a favorable approach in us, no matter what your condition may be.

With enhanced physical vitality, enhanced health and relief from stress and anxiety, Tourmaline stimulates our greater impulses, improving altruism and creativity.

Spiritual Healing

The main impact of Tourmaline is the balancing and grounding of our spiritual forces, enabling us to bring inspiration and energy into our daily life.

By activating the roots of our Root Chakra, Tourmaline aligns our etheric energy organs with Earth's components.

Tourmaline has the power to raise our frequency when we are in a negative state of mind and lighten our mood when we feel bleak, assisting us in staying light-hearted and safe.

Rare natural Tourmaline Wands are impregnated with unique energies that enable us to touch and even channel greater spiritual forces, creating incredible healing.

This powerful crystal can release blockages, clean the aura and purify our bodies from negative energies as well as protecting us against occult attacks.

Tourmaline Wands, placed in our feet or knee areas and facing back, have the potential to push adverse forces away.

They can also be utilized to guide the energies through the Crown Chakra, creating a perfect connection between the etheric body and the power meridians of the brain.

Tourmaline Crystal Uses

Tourmaline Crystals are frequently used by shamans for their vigorous and mystical characteristics, including as screeching rocks and as protective crystals during ceremonies.

Tourmaline has traditionally been used to disclose the cause of issues or the identity of the offender and may demonstrate the correct path to take in challenging moments.

Creating a ring of 8 tiny natural Tourmaline Stones functions as a protective circle in which healing rites can be performed and meditated.

Black Tourmaline is ideal for individual that experience emotional distress, assisting to manage our worries and to stay calm in confined spaces.

Those who fear Doctors and Dentists may use Tourmaline to quench their concerns and stay calm during medical trips and processes.

Tourmaline Crystals protect us from all types of negativity, particularly from those whose adverse behaviors are contagious, such as whiners, complainers and gossips.

Carrying a Tourmaline amulet or carrying a Tourmaline necklace can safeguard us from the bad vibrations emanated by emotional vampires.

Students may use Tourmaline Crystals to enhance concentration. When you feel dispersed and distracted, keep a piece of Black Tourmaline in your palm and breathe profoundly.

Tourmaline functions as a natural shield against damaging and toxic energy from cell phones, electronics, pcs and environmental pollutants.

Tourmaline Crystals can accompany us at our workplace, helping us remain grounded, conscious and effective.

Tourmaline Crystals are very strong, absorbing high-frequency vibrations of TV signals, radio signals and other vibrational models without breaking.

Tourmaline increases the workings of our senses, rendering them smooth and vibrant and may also have an aphrodisiac impact on those who perform them.

The strong, earthing energy that characterizes Tourmaline has the ability of diminishing and even annihilating motion sickness

Meditation with Tourmaline

Among the most used stones to perform meditation with, is Black Tourmaline, recognized for its benefits on helping individuals reach perfect equilibrium.

The vibration of Tourmaline promotes practicality, stabilization and grounding, making it ideal for meditators who are susceptible to fancy journeys.

As a protective stone, the meditator can investigate the universe of the Spirit without fear of damage or threat.

Tourmaline is perfect for purifying your aura and clearing the field of your etheric body.

Tourmaline Crystals can assist anyone bases their meditation exercise by balancing our mental forces and by activating the force that resides in our Root Chakra.

Tourmaline Crystal Zodiac Sign

Tourmaline is linked to those born between September 23rd and October 22nd, making Tourmaline the Zodiac stone of Libra.

During this moment of the year, the vernal equinox happens, which means that day and night are completely balanced.

The only zodiac sign represented by an inanimate item, The Libra depicts equilibrium.

Tourmaline's ability to balance the vibrations of body, mind and spirit makes it a quintessential stone for Librans who are willing, sensitive and creative.

Tourmaline's grounding and stabilizing power enables those using it to be more conscious, less challenging and more friendly.

Tourmaline Crystal Chakra

This crystal is often used to stimulate the energy of the base Chakra and align our root Chakra with the center of the Earth, forming a solid basis for our wellness and well-being.

The root Chakra, situated at the bottom of our spine, is the basis of our physical and mental power scheme.

By washing our root Chakra, Tourmaline stimulates our energy system, rouses us from lethargy and poor energy and relieves us from the need for incessant stimuli.

When our religious forces are out of tune and we feel confused and fugitive, carrying our Tourmaline grounds, assisting us to communicate profoundly with the globe around us.

When the Root Chakra is in equilibrium and aligned with our inner forces, the physical body receives energy and stamina.

Spiritual energy is being reintroduced and we feel safe and stable in the ownership of our power.

Tourmaline Amulets and Talismans

In old times, Tourmaline was regarded as the rock of the autumn and the gem of the evening.

The energy of Tourmaline guides us in the path of our greatest self, guiding us in the path of our power.

As an energizing glass, Tourmaline enables us to concentrate our energies and strengthen our life strength, assisting us in attaining our objectives.

By energizing us and assisting us to discover what we are looking for in this existence, Tourmaline preserves what we value and defends us from undesirable results that we expect to prevent.

CONCLUSION

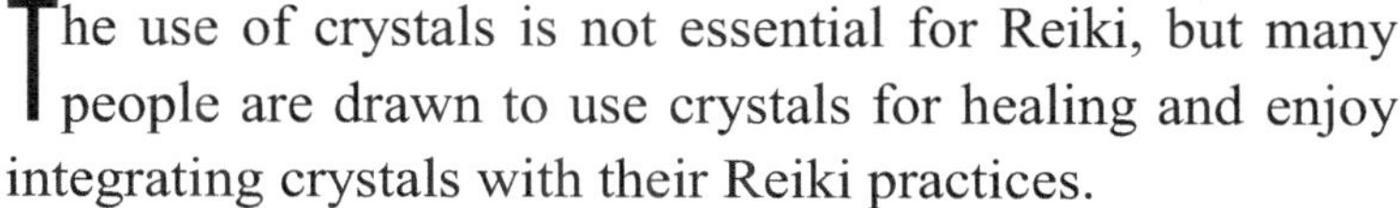

The use of crystals is not essential for Reiki, but many people are drawn to use crystals for healing and enjoy integrating crystals with their Reiki practices.

In crystal healing, we use crystals or gemstones for healing purposes. These gemstones are utilized to either cure physical discomfort or to purify the body from any contamination.

There are seven main regions in our bodies, known as "Chakras", so crystal healing procedures focus on these areas. In Hindi, the word "Chakra" means spiritual energy.

The main Chakras are described as our energy centers. As we saw earlier, crystals come in a wide variety of shapes and colors and every color has a different significance and importance.

The energy flows through our Chakras, purifying our bodies. Crystal healing helps us to achieve equilibrium. The healer who performs the process on someone needs to start by undergoing a mending procedure on himself, in order to get rid of any eventual negative energy. This energy can then be transferred between the bodies through the crystals. By doing so, the person affected by any harmful vibration will be healed.

Crystal healing has gained a great amount of popularity today, not only between individuals suffering from illnesses of some kind. Placing crystals directly on the energy centers is not mandatory. These precious stones are also helpful when kept close to the bed at night, or in a study room and they can be worn as talismans. The crystal use varies based on the disturbance an individual might suffer from or depending on the energy one wants to clear or revive.

We do not possess a solid knowledge of how crystal healing started as a practice. People have been using it for thousands of years. We know that our ancestors didn't have much faith in crystal healing and the majority of people supposed it was spiritual. But we are now witnessing a big change in how individuals perceive crystal healing as many have started to understand the impact of this practice. Although it is not scientifically proven that crystal healing works, only those who have undergone such sessions know its actual power.

Due to its color and shape, the majority of crystal healers practice with the help of clear quartz. But different stones work for different reasons.

Is there any harm to healing? The practice itself is not harmful in any way. But every individual needs to know that crystal healing is not an alternative to medication, so no one should ever give up on medical treatment in favor of this practice. In many religions it is thought that if the wrong energy is carried through during crystal healing, it may be very dangerous, since these forces that are transmitted are not connected to God and therefore can be very hazardous.

Benefits Crystal Give You

Several advantages that assist the spiritual development of an individual, as well as mental and physical ailments. Some of the strongest advantages of crystal healing are the use of crystal therapy for personal development, wellness and vitality. Healers work with you in order to stimulate changes within yourself, to liberate your mind from any harmful energy and to help curing physical conditions when traditional medicine doesn't seem to work or requires to be coupled with holistic methods to stimulate rehabilitation. Crystals are also amazing for individuals experiencing anxiety and depression, for people who are under a lot of stress or just for those who want to relax and relieve themselves of any negativity. They can assist with menstrual issues, headaches, digestive issues, pain relief, fatigue, memory loss, concentration and even teaching difficulties. It has shown excellent outcomes in relationship construction, property building and private self-fulfillment.

It advantages the environment by combining the mind with the mood that balances the environment. It can stimulate creativity, enhance communication and even assist in developing your spirituality. It is not suggested that you substitute medical therapy if it is required, but it can offer a boost to your well-being that can genuinely enhance your body and mind. From enhancing emotions of empowerment, inspirational love, or relieving migraines, healers give a universe of advantages to anyone